About the Authors

LANI LOPEZ is one of New Zealand's leading qualified naturopaths. She has over 16 years' experience in the field of natural medicine and contributes regularly to radio and television. Lani has been the supplement researcher and designer for Good Health Products for the last nine years and she also presents lectures and seminars for the natural food and supplement industry. Qualified as a naturopath, Lani also has a basic knowledge of Indonesian herbal medicine and a little of Ayurvedic (Indian) herbal medicine. Her first book, *Natural Health – an A to Z Guide*, was published in October 2004.

JENNA MOORE was the beauty and wellbeing editor of *Next* magazine for eight years before 'going solo' at the end of 2004. She has over 20 years experience in the beauty and wellness industry. Over time her journalistic contribution to *Next* magazine widened to include her special interest in health and the empowerment of women. She created and edited the annual Breast Cancer Special Report which was first published in 2000 and she has spent over five years extensively researching breast cancer.

Lani and Jenna met while judging Miss Auckland in 2000 along with a young woman named Jo Sutherland. A previous Miss Auckland contestant, Jo had been diagnosed with breast cancer at the age of 28. She died in May 2003 at just 31 and has left a large void in many people's lives. Jo's beauty and *joie de vivre* were enjoyed by many people and her illness was the impetus for this book. Jo brought Lani and Jenna together and her influence caused them to discover a mutual passion for reducing ignorance about breast cancer, particularly in younger women. Younger women are usually not aware they can develop the disease but, although it's rare, they can and do. It is not by any means a probability – the majority of women diagnosed with breast cancer are over 50 – however, Lani and Jenna feel strongly that younger women must know their youth doesn't automatically make them immune. If you are pre-menopausal the disease is more aggressive, so the earlier it is detected the more chance there is of controlling it.

In the pink

A guide to breasts, cancer and living well

Lani Lopez & Jenna Moore

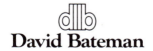

Disclaimer: The information in this book does not constitute medical advice. It should not be used as a manual for self-treatment. The information herein was compiled to help you make informed choices about your health. The publisher and writers cannot guarantee the safety or effectiveness of any drug, treatment or advice mentioned. We recommend in all cases that you should consult a licensed professional healthcare provider before taking or discontinuing any medications or before treating yourself in any way. It is recommended you consult with your GP when looking at lifestyle changes, particularly if you have a medical condition. Herbs and some medications can interact. Please check with your doctor first. If you are pregnant or breastfeeding, see your health professional for advice before starting any health programmes. Do not come off prescription medication.

Copyright © Lani Lopez and Jenna Moore, 2005
Copyright © David Bateman Ltd, 2005

First published 2005 by David Bateman Ltd,
30 Tarndale Grove, Albany, Auckland, New Zealand

ISBN 1-86953-609-6

This book is copyright. Except for the purpose of fair review, no part may be stored or transmitted in any form or by any means, electronic or mechanical, including recording or storage in any information retrieval systems, without permission in writing from the publisher. No reproduction may be made, whether by photocopying or by any other means, unless a licence has been obtained from the publisher or its agent.

Cover photography by Sally Tagg
Model: Victoria Lovrich; Body painting, hair and makeup by Nikki Lovrich
Backdrop from Global Fabrics; Flowers by Urban Flowers
Authors' makeup by Shonagh Murray using Estée Lauder makeup
Design by Alice Bell
Printed in China through Everbest Printing Company Ltd.

Dedication

We dedicate this book with love and loads of bee kisses to Jo Sutherland. You know what we mean when we say, we hope you're dancing.

A Jo quote: 'Think before you speak. Anyone you see could have breast cancer. Most of us look vibrant and healthy.'

Contents

Acknowledgements	8
Foreword	11
A letter to our readers	12
1: Examining the breast	17
2: About breast cancer	25
3: On treatment	37
4: Exploring the side effects of having breast cancer	59
5: What you can do to reduce the risk of getting breast cancer	81
6: Mind–body healing	105
7: Looking to the future	127
Services and contacts	130
Further reading to help you through	132
Useful websites	134
Endnotes	135
Bibliography	142
Index	143

Acknowledgements

WE'D LIKE TO THANK our publisher David Bateman Ltd, particularly Paul Bateman for seeing the value in this book, Tracey Borgfeldt for her wonderful patience and lovely manner, Andrea Hassall for putting it all together, and Tim Brown (our publicist) and Bryce Gibson for helping to get our message out there.

LANI would particularly like to thank: Belinda Hope-Too who graciously lent me her New Zealand nutritional research paper on 'The role of nutritional supplements in cancer' – it gave me the courage to write this book; Steve Charnley – all-round good guy, soul mate and great husband. Thanks for making me laugh when the going got a bit tough. That's one of the many reasons I love being with you; Jessica and James Charnley – thank you for all your support and love. You mean the entire world to me. I'm glad to be part of your lives; Tracey Borgfeldt – I couldn't have finished this without you as my editor. This has certainly been one of the most challenging projects I've ever had to complete; my family and friends – writing takes a fair bit of social sacrifice. Thanks for waiting for me; and Jenna – the work you have done is exquisite and I am completely humbled.

JENNA would particularly like to thank: June Nevin, without her generosity my contribution would never have been possible; Liz Parker, former editor of *Next* magazine, for seeing the value of informing New Zealanders about breast cancer and for being there when the going got rough (as it so often did!); Jo Sutherland, Reigan Allan and Wendy Claughton for allowing me to learn with them about the journey of breast cancer during their too short lives; Dr Nicole McCarthy for her enthusiasm in improving breast cancer treatment in New Zealand and for taking the time to check my medical facts. (Nicole is a breast cancer researcher at the University of Auckland and the medical oncologist at Auckland Hospital. Her work is partly funded by the proceeds from the Glassons breast cancer t-shirts – so keep buying them!); all of the doctors, surgeons, oncologists, radiotherapists and other specialists who have shared their time and expertise over the years – Mr Janek Januszkiewicz, Dr Belinda Scott, Mr John Harman, Dr Richard Harman, Mr Trevor Smith, Dr Vernon Harvey and Dr Benji Benjamin; the wonderful people who have shared their stories with me – you all know who you are and I am very grateful to have met you; Cate Carden, I hope I am saying just a little of what you would like to; Dr John Link for introducing me to an American contingent of medical specialists who were extraordinarily generous with their knowledge; Dr Link's sister Debbie and her family for sharing their story, and the entire family for welcoming me into their homes in Auckland and Los Angeles; Russell Moore (my brother) for looking after Cassidy while I was gone; Leslie Kenton, Tina-Marie Sharman, Cecilie Geary, Marama Brown, Claire McCall, Hilary Timmins, Sarah Paykel, Sally Davies, Trina and Krista Verdonk, Zara Atkinson, Eadon Howe, Sue Giddens and so many more wonderful people who have given me professional feedback, support and believed in me; Mrs Evelyn Lauder who (quite unknowingly) inspired me to make the break and give it a go; Sally Tagg for her beautiful photography; Nikki Lovrich for her wonderful body-painting for our cover and her beautiful sister Victoria for being our model; and, of course, I must thank Lani Lopez for being such an inspirational friend and for prodding me in the back!

Foreword

I AM HONOURED to write a foreword to this excellent book, a book that will give women important knowledge and practical information about breast cancer. As a breast cancer doctor and researcher for over twenty years, it is clear to me that knowledge is power. Women who partner with their medical team and 'engage' in a plan that includes the best modern medicine has to offer along with complementary therapy for the 'mind, body and soul', have better outcomes and quality of life.

The world is shrinking and information abounds. The crisis of breast cancer requires a woman to become educated quickly to make important treatment decisions. A major problem is what information is accurate, helpful and trustworthy. It has been one of my professional goals to help women in this regard with my own books and internet information site 'breastlink.com'. This book is a wonderful addition to that goal of helping women to become informed in a partnership with their healers.

No one goes untouched by breast cancer. It is all around us. Fortunately, women have better chances for cure because of earlier diagnosis and more effective treatment. My own sister developed breast cancer five years ago in New Zealand. With intensive pre-surgical chemotherapy, she had a complete response and, at the time of her surgery, there was no remaining disease in her breast or lymph nodes.

Technology is giving us new treatments and diagnostic tools. It is important to prove them beneficial and allow women access to them in a timely manner. If possible, women should enrol in research trials because it is the only way to prove a treatment helps. It is also a way of helping women in the future who develop this disease.

Lastly, as a physician I am so appreciative to the women with this disease – it is truly an honour to witness their courage, honesty, openness and generosity. For those of you beginning this book, one undeserved journey of breast cancer, I wish you well.

Dr John Link M.D.
Breast Oncologist
Medical Director Breastlink Medical Group
Director Long Beach Memorial Breast Cancer Center

A letter to our readers

WE WANTED TO write this book to offer a user-friendly, down-to-earth guide that's readily available to the women (and men*), and their friends and family, who are diagnosed with breast cancer each year. We are not medical doctors nor have we experienced breast cancer ourselves, however, through our professions, we have had close contact with many people who have. Women are terrified of the words breast cancer and many of them choose to block out its existence, but could we take a moment to share with you a lesson we have learned? Knowledge gives power, understanding gives power and information gives power. Becoming informed about your body is paramount to good health. Breast cancer has a negative image and many people equate it with a death sentence. THIS DOES NOT HAVE TO BE SO! Breast cancer doesn't necessarily mean death or even the loss of a breast but sometimes, when the words relate to yourself or someone close to you, that's a little hard to grasp. If you are hit closely by the disease it can be mind-blowingly overwhelming. We've tried to simplify the initial information process and answer the questions you probably don't have your head together enough to ask. We've added a few thought-provoking theories, beneficial holistic techniques and Lani has provided from her extensive knowledge of natural therapies some tools you can feel comfortable using. None of the methods we explore are meant to take the place of traditional medicine, they are tools that anyone can use for general wellbeing but are not proven cures for disease. Well, not as far as we know anyway.

Our message to you is, please, don't hide your head in the sand. Feel your breasts, become familiar with them and realise that if they feel different it's probably nothing. Nine times out of ten any breast abnormality won't be cancerous. If you feel something is not right and your doctor tells you to wait and see, get a second opinion and even a third opinion. If nothing is wrong, great. But if it turns out to be cancerous at least you've found out and you can take action. Ignoring it won't make it go away!

This advice applies whatever your age. In the past I (Jenna) have been much maligned for trying to increase the awareness of breast cancer in younger women. My intention was not to scaremonger or misrepresent the statistics but I feel strongly that youth shouldn't bypass awareness. International pop diva Anastacia has launched a trust to increase awareness in women under 40 after undergoing a lumpectomy, reconstructive surgery and radiotherapy treatment. Her message is 'give up that pair of shoes, don't go out for that expensive dinner – get a mammogram'. (Of course, that may be difficult if you can't afford the shoes or the dinner in the first place, but you get the drift.) Which brings us to the ongoing argument. Mammograms aren't infallible and it's hard to read younger women's breasts as the tissue is denser and can camouflage a tumour (see page 21). No one can argue with that, but using ultrasound in conjunction with a mammogram can increase the odds of an accurate reading. Let's not blow the matter out of all proportion, just becoming familiar with your breasts helps and if you have particular concerns have a medical check – think of it as part of your personal warrant of fitness. You have a regular smear test and dental examination, don't you?

In essence this book is about breasts and living well. We've combined our different areas of expertise to bring you an informative book that's an easy read (we hope) not a medical tome. It's our heartfelt wish that the words printed on these pages are of benefit to you or someone you love. And we hope they provide more comfort than fear. We don't claim to have all the answers, but it's our sincere desire that this book will offer useful information and advice that won't clog your brain cells. If you want a more comprehensive guide look for *Dr Susan Love's Breast Book* or Dr John Link's *The Breast Cancer Survival Manual* – they cover everything, and we mean everything, you need to know.

---

* One per cent of those diagnosed with breast cancer each year are men. However, for the purposes of convenience we have used women as a reference.

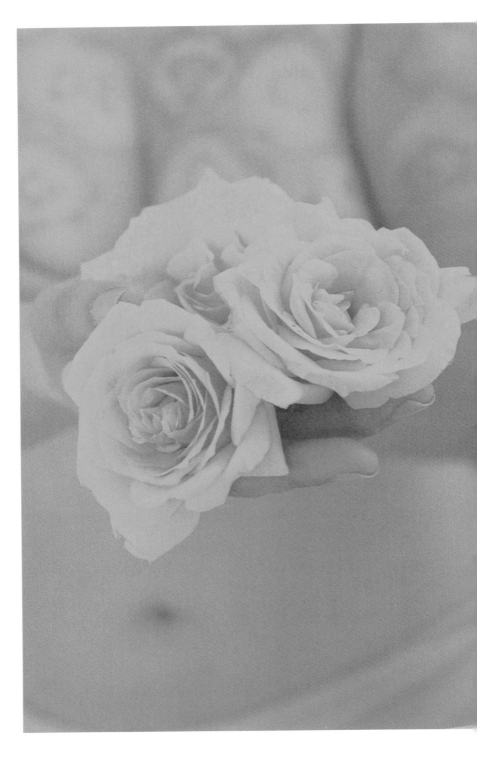

Unforgettable

She is a mother who can think only of the welfare of her children.
She is a wife who wonders if her husband will still love her.
She is a daughter horrified of the thought of breaking the news to her ageing parents.
She is a sister, a soulmate, the best girl you know.
She is a friend, a real bosom buddy.
She is a neighbour who now needs a friend.
She is an executive who has lost her control.
She is an employee who wonders how she will keep her job, pay her bills, take care of her child, while trying to recover.
She is a patient who fears losing her life.
She is a doctor who must now save her own life.
She is a beauty who now feels like a beast.
She is a beast who never did feel beautiful.
She is famous and now wishes she wasn't.
She is a stranger who you can't see, but she can see you.
She is a person whom you have yet to meet.
She is you, she is me,
She is …. Unforgettable

In honour and remembrance of all who have survived, battled or lost the fight against breast cancer by Cristina Carlino (creator of Philosophy Skincare).

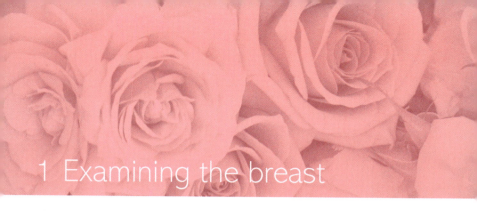

1 Examining the breast

Breasts, boobs, bazookas, mammary glands: we know we've got them, but what exactly are they?

DO YOU REMEMBER when your first swollen mosquito bites (aka breasts) started to appear? Most of us found it exciting (OK tomboys, maybe not you), even if it hurt a bit. These little beauties, along with our galloping hormones, underarm and pubic threads, were a sign we were, at long last, growing up. The finished result, i.e., the shape and size of your adult breasts, is largely determined by genetics although the size will vary with pregnancy and weight gain.

Whatever size you've inherited – delicate buds or a substantial handful – your breasts will be made up of glandular, fatty and fibrous (connective) tissues – about one third fat and two thirds other tissue. The fat is what makes the breasts feel soft. You'll also have a pair of nipples which can be perky, slight or inverted and they will be surrounded by a roundish-shaped area called the areola. The nipples and areola tend to be pink or brownish in colour and darken during orgasm and pregnancy. Both contain small sphincter-like muscles which cause the areola to pucker and the nipple to rise in cold weather and during sexual arousal. The areola is also home to hair follicles so the odd hair is not uncommon (if you don't like this you can easily remove them by plucking or electrolysis). You may also notice a collection of 'bumps' here. These are called Montgomery glands and help with lubrication – if you've ever experienced dry or cracked nipples you'll understand the importance of this function.

Along with these aesthetic characteristics are the internal elements that run throughout the entire body such as veins, arteries and lymph vessels. The arteries carry blood rich with oxygen from the heart to the cells of the chest wall and breasts, and the veins carry the oxygen-depleted blood full of carbon dioxide back to the heart. The lymph vessels remove any waste products (more about the lymphatic system later).

The primary role of the breasts (apart from sexual pleasure) is milk production. Breasts house the lobules – glands that produce milk – and the ductal system – the system through which the milk travels. During breastfeeding (lactation) the lobules swing into action turning blood into the milk that travels through the ducts to the nipple to be suckled by the baby.[1]

THE BREAST
Typical lymph node sites that can be involved in cancer development.

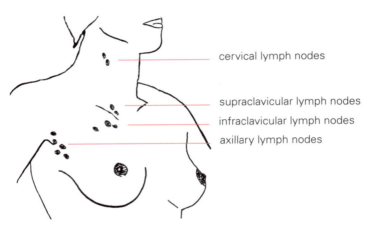

Structure of mammary glands and the breast.

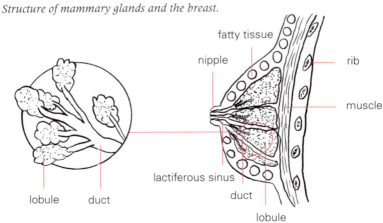

1 | EXAMINING THE BREAST

Getting to know you

How often have you taken the time to become familiar with your breasts? Possibly your lover/partner/husband knows more about their shape and feel than you do. There is a trend in our society that it's 'wrong' to feel our bodies, particularly our erogenous zones. Dr Susan Love advocates getting familiar with our own breasts in her book – *Dr Susan Love's Breast Book*. Dr Love has studied the breast and has treated breast disease for many years and her opinion is well respected. She doesn't advocate the controversial breast self-examination (BSE) as she feels this practice encourages us to look for our body to betray us.[2] We agree. However, we'd like to say that that doesn't mean BSE isn't a useful tool. What is important is your attitude. If you practise BSE with a mental attitude the same as you have when you're taking your car for a warrant of fitness (as we talked about earlier), you'll keep in perspective the worry of any serious disease lurking. By getting to know your breasts you're not actively looking for something to be wrong, you're simply becoming familiar with your own body. Take the time to look in the mirror at your breasts, cup them, knead them, feel how sensitive (or not) they are. Do the same in the shower or bath when they're all soapy – they could very well feel different again. Lift your arm behind your head. Change position. Doing this at different times of the month you'll see how they can change with your cycle (if you're pre-menopausal and not taking hormones). The amount of fat in your breast can make them feel soft and springy and you may even feel your ribcage at some stage. If you feel a lump or see an indentation chances are it's not breast cancer. Even some nipple discharge is not uncommon. Some women can experience discharge when their breast is squeezed. But it's only by knowing your own breasts that you'll recognise any significant changes.

BREAST SELF-EXAMINATION: THE STEPS

1. Stand in front of a mirror, place your hands at your sides. Check your breasts for any lumps, changes in colour or shape, any rashes or scaling, dimpling or puckering, inverted nipples or nipple discharge.
2. Check again in the mirror. This time raise both arms. After this, place your hands on your hips and press shoulders and elbows forward to flex your chest muscles. Look for any changes as noted above.
3. Lie down and perform a physical examination. Raise one arm and use a flat palm and the balls of your three middle fingers. Move in circles and spirals around the breast. Do the same with the other breast and don't forget to check under and below your armpits.[3]

Something's different...what now?

First of all, don't panic. That may sound trite because it's only natural you will worry. But please remember that nine out of ten breast lumps, indentations and other changes are not cancerous. Most early breast cancer has no symptoms. Benign (which means harmless) changes are quite common so immediately jumping to conclusions will only cause you undue angst. Lumpiness (as opposed to a single, more prominent lump) can often appear around the time of your period. Also fibroadenomas (smooth, round, hard lumps), cysts (fluid-filled sacs) and connective tissue hyperplasia (enlarged glands) are not uncommon and will often manifest as a lump or unusual area that's harmless. Mastalgia (breast pain) can also occur and is often related to hormonal changes. Even a nipple discharge may not mean anything more serious than a benign growth inside the breast. (About one per cent of discharges are cancerous.) A certain amount of nipple discharge (thick, white/yellowish) is considered quite normal. However, it is not normal if the discharge is bloody or watery. Even though symptoms like these are probably harmless you still need to make an appointment with your doctor. They should listen to your symptoms and concerns, give you a clinical examination, possibly send you for a mammogram and ultrasound and maybe perform a biopsy. If they don't take you seriously, go to someone else. Making light of your concerns is unacceptable.

A word about hormonally lumpy breasts

'Don't touch my breasts! You can look, but don't touch.' Do these words sometimes go through your mind? Most women can empathise with others when their breasts become a little lumpier, tender and larger in response to hormone fluctuations. This is quite normal.

Your breasts may swell, feel tender and have little nodules just before or during menstruation which then disappear afterwards. Although some research conflicts with the idea that natural remedies work for women with lumpy breasts, many anecdotal reports and some supportive research suggest that dietary restriction and supplements can reduce pain, water retention and lumpy, tender breasts.[4,5,6,7,8] Take evening primrose oil (3000mg) with fish oil capsules (3000mg), natural vitamin E (400IU) and a vitamin B complex daily for 7–10 days leading up to menstruation and, if needed, five days during menstruation.

Reducing salt intake and avoiding coffee during this time may also help reduce water retention. If you do have lumpy breasts, either premenstrually, all the time or after menopause, tell your health professional. If necessary they'll suggest a breast examination. This will let you know what is going on hormonally with your breasts and what you can do about it.

POULTICE HERBS FOR BREAST INFLAMMATION, NIPPLE DISCHARGE AND CYSTS

Poultices can help with breast seepage, breast cysts and inflammation of the breasts. A handful of fresh, whole bruised or crushed comfrey or yellow dock leaves and a grated raw potato can be mixed together, contained in a muslin cloth or bag and placed on the affected breast or nipple. This is a very drawing poultice recipe and can be used up to three times daily. Leave on the breast for 30 minutes then discard. Make a fresh poultice per application.

What happens at the doctor's office?

There are typically two scenarios you'll encounter here. (Thankfully the latter option occurs less and less.) For whatever reason, you present at your GP with a concern about your breasts. Your doctor will either listen to your concerns, perform a clinical examination and then send you off for a mammogram and/or ultrasound or they will tell you to wait a period of time and see what happens. If you experience the latter, get a second opinion. Women are notorious for not standing up for themselves. Trust your instincts.

WHAT IS A MAMMOGRAM?

A mammogram is a low dose x-ray of the breast. It has gained a bad reputation as being uncomfortable and even painful because it squashes the breast between two plates, like a sandwich. Most operators are sensitive to your needs and if you avoid pre-menstrual times or other occasions when your breasts are sensitive you shouldn't experience too much discomfort. Small breasted women complain it's uncomfortable more than larger breasted women, which makes sense. They haven't got as much breast fat and tissue to make the sandwich with, so they may experience a bit more pulling and prodding. Even so, most women agree they much prefer undergoing a mammogram than a pap smear! Feelings aside, breast cancer specialists say a mammogram is currently the best means we have to detect breast cancer. However, it is also universally agreed it's not a perfect method and will miss 10 to 15 per cent of breast cancers. An infallible method of detection has yet to be created (be assured though, people are working on it).

Mammography works better on some women than others. If you have dense breast tissue, as younger women and women on hormone replacement therapy typically do, your x-ray will be more difficult to read. Dense breast tissue shows opaque white on a mammogram. Fat appears translucent black. Any tumours or other abnormalities show up as white through the black. Hence, if the breast is dense it can be like looking for a sandhopper on the beach.

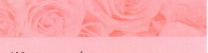

In adolescence, when women first evolve, they begin to develop breast tissue. As women age, this tissue turns to fat. So, in mammogram terms, over time the breast shows more and more translucent black and it's easier to see abnormalities. Of course there are exceptions to every rule and some women keep their breast density as they age. And some tumours are just plain difficult to read.

In New Zealand, mammography is funded by the government for women aged 45–69.

> When you go for a mammogram you will be asked to remove your clothes to the waist and don a medical gown, so it is best to wear a skirt or pants and a top. Also avoid deodorant, talcum powder and fragrance as any residue can interfere with the film. (This is probably advisable for all screening methods.) A new study shows breast cancers detected by screening mammography are more likely to be treated with breast conservation and without chemotherapy.[9]

WHAT IS AN ULTRASOUND?

Ultrasound is often used in conjunction with mammography for younger women with dense breasts and when an abnormality can be felt in the breast but does not show up on a mammogram. Ultrasound works by the use of high-frequency sound waves (which is hard for people like you and me to fathom) transmitted into a precise body area. Basically, it's just like the ultrasound used in pregnancy. A gel is applied to the breast area and a hand-held probe is moved across the skin and the sound waves go through the breast. The waves echo back to the computer and are converted into an image. Whereas on a mammogram breast density and abnormalities show up white, on ultrasound the density still shows white but any abnormality shows up black. Breast specialists say ultrasound is an extremely useful tool because it enables them to get a lot of information very quickly. In seconds they will know whether they are dealing with a simple fluid-filled cyst or a harder lump. And when ultrasound is used in conjunction with biopsy it helps locate the exact area to be biopsied (see page 24). There is no hit and miss aspect. However, ultrasound readings are very operator dependent so it's important that the person who does the reading is experienced.

WHAT IS THERMOGRAPHY?

Thermography, as a screening tool for breast cancer, is based on the theory that cancer gives off heat. A device is put over the breast and a very pretty blue and red picture is created on a screen. Blue registers cold, red registers hot. It's very sensitive, and therefore, can pick up all manner of things in the breast. Experts say the problem is that it picks up too much and has proved to be inaccurate. On the other hand, if a breast cancer sits deeply in the breast it is less likely to be picked up at all. Recently this technique has been the subject of media focus again in the form of advertising and advertorials, but most breast specialists don't feel it has a place in screening as it is not specific enough and can put people through unnecessary stress and worry. The New Zealand Breast Cancer Foundation advise only using it as a screening tool in conjunction with mammography.

WHAT IS MRI (MAGNETIC RESONANCE IMAGING)?

An MRI is a scan that can be used to view cross sections of parts of the body. In the case of breast cancer this is, of course, the breast. The scan works rather like an angiogram. A dye (called contrast medium) is injected into the veins and travels through the body. The dye is picked up by soft tissues, particularly those with lots of blood vessels (a common characteristic of some cancer tumours). This shows as a picture on the machine's computer screen and enables the operator to get a clear view, from many angles, of the tumour. The pictures show exactly where and what size a tumour is. MRI scans are sensitive and can be as much as 99 per cent accurate. However, the technology is only used in special cases in this country as it is very expensive (around $700–$1,000 per session). 'Special cases' may include women at high-risk of getting breast cancer, incidents when there is a known cancer, and when other methods of scanning, such as mammogram or ultrasound, are difficult to read, for example, if the woman has very dense breast tissue or scarring from radiation or surgery. It is also commonly used for women with breast implants.

WHAT IS A BIOPSY?

If a suspicious area or lump is diagnosed or found after a routine screening you will probably be asked to undergo a biopsy. There are a few types of biopsy and which one you undergo will depend on the signs and symptoms you are showing. The good news is that 80 per cent of biopsy results aren't cancerous. In simple terms, a biopsy is an examination of a sample of abnormal tissue and it is the only way to tell if cancer is present. It can also show what type of cancer has reared its head and how fast it is growing. A needle is used to extract tissue from the suspicious area and the specimen is smeared onto a glass slide whereupon it goes to a pathologist to be read under a microscope.

• **Fine aspiration:** A very, very fine needle is inserted into the lump and a small amount of fluid and cells are drawn out.
• **Core biopsy:** This requires a slightly bigger needle (though not a big, thick plunger) and a 'worm' of tissue is extracted. This is sliced finely and placed on a slide.
• **Core biopsy – stereotactic:** This is the same process as above but a special apparatus also gives the radiologists/pathologists a 3D image.
• **Exicisional surgical biopsy:** The lump or mass as well as a surrounding margin of normal tissue is removed. This procedure is done under local anaesthetic and is more frequently used for harmless (benign) lesions.
• **Wire localisation biopsy:** Sometimes an abnormality can be seen by mammography or ultrasound but it can't be felt. The ultrasound machine can be very helpful here as a guidance tool. Using the screen as a visual guide, a radiologist inserts very fine stainless-steel wires into the suspicious area. These act as a placement guide for the surgeon to help ensure the right area is excised.

A recent study found that anxiety medication may be useful for women preparing to undergo biopsy. Dr Lawrence Bassett, from the University of California in Los Angeles, and colleagues found that women treated with an anxiety-relieving drug 15 minutes before the procedure had a 44 per cent decrease in stress levels.[10]

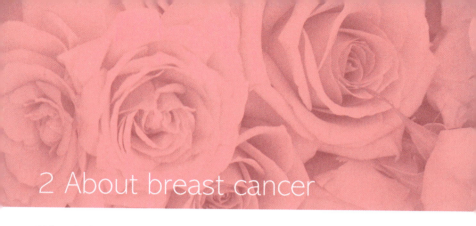

2 About breast cancer

What is breast cancer?

THE BODY IS a complex thing and to understand breast cancer you'd need to be *au fait* with the molecular biology of it. Most of us don't want, or indeed need, to go that far. Following is a very simple explanation of the disease.

Our bodies are made up of millions of cells which divide and reproduce constantly. The trouble starts when one of these cells mutates and keeps on dividing uncontrollably. Breast tumours are caused by a cell, usually located in the breast ducts or, in some cases, the lobules, which acts like a 'villain' who's champing at the bit to cause some trouble. The villain has the ability to divide and multiply into clones of itself until it rages out of control and uses the combined power of its multiple selves to wreak havoc in the rest of the body.

However, while it's on its rampage, if it manages to enter the lymphatic system it'll come up against fierce opposition. You see, it'll start swimming in lymph fluid whose main purpose is to get rid of foreign invaders like the villain. And if it manages to outwit the fluid and infiltrates the lymph nodes, they'll register it in the unwanted fluid and then it'll be in serious trouble.

Lymph nodes are small bean-shaped collections of immune system cells called lymphocytes and they are specifically programmed to trap and destroy cancer cells. So, because they know the villain is intent on causing harm, they will hold on to it while they develop an antibody to neutralise it. This is why sometimes your lymph nodes will swell when you have an infection. They're fighting to overpower the danger. But, and here's the worry, if the original villain is strong enough, it will overpower the lymph node and continue to grow in power. This is where the villain gets really scary.

Types of breast cancer

Most cancers manifest as a single, hard, non-movable, non-tender lump in one breast. However, cancers that are situated deep in the breast may pull the ligament which gives them the appearance of an indentation rather than a lump.

In situ is the term used for the early stage of cancer, when it is confined to the immediate area where it began. Specifically in breast cancer, *in situ* means that the cancer remains confined to ducts (ductal carcinoma *in situ*) or lobules (lobular carcinoma *in situ*). It has not invaded surrounding tissues in the breast nor spread to other organs in the body. Eighty-five per cent of tumours will occur in the duct and 15 per cent in the lobules.

- **Ductal carcinoma *in situ* (DCIS):** DCIS is the most common type of non-invasive breast cancer. It means the cancer cells have developed inside the ducts but have not spread through the walls of the ducts into the surrounding breast tissue. This is completely curable.
- **Lobular carcinoma *in situ* (LCIS):** Although not a true cancer, LCIS is sometimes classified as a type of non-invasive breast cancer. It begins in the milk-producing glands but does not penetrate through the wall of the lobules. Women with LCIS need to pay close attention to screening.
- **Invasive (infiltrating) ductal carcinoma (IDC):** This is the most common type of breast cancer. The cancer starts in a duct of the breast and invades through the duct into the surrounding tissues. If it's strong enough it can spread to other parts of the body. (This is the only type of breast cancer that occurs in men.)
- **Invasive (infiltrating) lobular carcinoma (ILC):** The cancer starts in the milk-producing glands, or lobules, and can also invade through the lobules and spread to other parts of the body. This type of cancer isn't as detectable by mammogram as IDC.

There are some other types of breast cancers that are uncommon:

- **Medullary carcinoma:** This type of tumour often has a clear boundary between it and normal tissue, it has a better prognosis than some other types of breast cancer.
- **Mucinous carcinoma:** This type is invasive and formed by mucous-producing cancer cells. It also has a better prognosis than some of the other types of breast cancer.
- **Tubular carcinoma:** This type of cancer is less likely to have spread when it is found and has quite a good prognosis.
- **Inflammatory breast cancer:** The skin of the breast may look red and

thick and feel warm, and is often mistaken for an infection and treated with antibiotics initially. This is the most aggressive type of breast cancer and is associated with a poorer prognosis.
• **Paget's disease of the nipple:** The tumour starts in the duct but spreads to the nipple and areola area. It can manifest on the skin around the nipple as scaly, red and crusty, and there may be bleeding, itching or burning.

In a separate category is the **Phyllodes tumour**: This very rare tumour develops in the connective tissue of the breast. It's usually benign (harmless) although it can be malignant.

METASTATIC DISEASE
Something a lot of people don't talk about is metastatic disease. It's kind of a taboo subject because it means the cancer has spread and become secondary cancer. People automatically assume this is a death sentence but, the good news is, this isn't a given. 'Metastatic disease is rarely curable but it's very treatable and women can live for many years with good quality of life,' says medical oncologist Dr Nicole McCarthy. Usually if breast cancer wants to travel to other parts of the body it chooses to go to the bones, liver, lungs or brain but once it gets there it may just sit for years and years, sometimes forever (presumably that ol' villain lies down and goes to sleep). Doctors hope that as medical knowledge about metastatic disease progresses – and it does every day – they will learn how to keep the cancer cells asleep indefinitely. The really important message here is that secondary breast cancer can be controlled and there are women out there going to the gym, taking their kids to school and doing all the normal things in life with metastatic breast cancer.

Who gets breast cancer?

Predominantly women, but one per cent of men are affected too. The incidence of breast cancer increases with age – women over 50 make up about 84 per cent of breast cancer sufferers. However, it is important to note that just because younger women make up only 15 or 16 per cent of the statistics it is 15 or 16 per cent too many. The 15 or 16 per cent I know all have names and families and wonderful spirits. There is a saying: 'Statistics are people without the tears.' And that pretty much says it all.

RISK FACTORS
RELATED TO AGE:
20s – 1 in 2500
30s – 1 in 232
40s – 1 in 55
50s – 1 in 40
60s – 1 in 29 [11]

WHAT IF I HAVE BREAST CANCER?

If you have the misfortune to get a positive diagnosis for cancer your world will turn upside down. Will I die? Will I lose my breast? Those questions will undoubtedly go through your mind constantly. You will probably only hear the word cancer and nothing more will swim through your mind for a time. You may cry or scream or go silent. Or all of the above. This is understandable. You are terrified. However, one thing breast cancer specialists will tell you is that you don't have to make treatment decisions immediately. You have some time. And you must know you are not alone. There are many, many organisations geared to help you and your loved ones so please, please, please get in touch with them (we've listed them at the back of this book). There are some pretty special and understanding people working in this field. You will be embarking on an enormous learning curve as the experience, treatment and molecular biology of breast cancer is complex and any support you and your friends and family can get will help you.

Without meaning to sound like Pollyanna you are being diagnosed with breast cancer in a time when knowledge and research has come a long way. The medical profession recognise the need to take into account both the mind and the body when it comes to illness. Breast cancer surgery is also called breast conservation surgery because the aim is to take as little of the breast as possible. If you must undergo surgery you won't have to 'go under' not knowing whether you will wake with a breast or not which used to be standard procedure in the past. And, if you choose to have reconstruction and it is the right choice for you, there are some mighty fine breast reconstructive surgeons who will work with you.

The Cancer Society provides invaluable counselling, transport services, meals, accommodation, information, library resources, aromatherapy, massage – a great number of services designed specifically for you and they've asked us to say right here, 'please use them'. It is our cherished hope that some of the tips and tools included in this book will help you on your journey also. Many of them are gleaned from women who have walked a similar path.

What causes breast cancer?

Nobody knows or fully understands the cause of breast cancer. As there are many sub-types of breast cancer the incidence is highly unlikely to have just one cause but it is becoming clear that modern life in Western society leads to increased risk. It is also widely believed to be the result of an overproduction of oestrogen in the body. (We manufacture our own oestrogen but certain foods, drugs, body types, chemicals and environmental factors can increase the levels.) Breast cancer is a multifactorial disease, that is, a disease where there is not one known factor but rather a combination of risk factors.[12,13] There are a couple of known causes and many causative theories abound. Of the known causes genetics are important, although not as common as is generally thought. Only five to ten per cent of breast cancers are family linked and genetic testing can help you determine this. Other factors believed to play a part in breast cancer diagnosis are: beginning menstruation later in life; having no pregnancies; a high calorie/fat diet; being overweight; a moderately high intake of alcohol (more than two glasses per day); lack of exercise; and exposure to radiation. The jury is still out on hormone medications, fertility drugs, pesticides and other environmental hazards, electromagnetic field exposure and being from a higher-socio economic background (presumably because you can afford access to the risk factors). These are discussed in more detail in the following pages.

'I think it's a combination of these factors that make up modern society,' says Mr Trevor Smith, breast specialist at Auckland's Ascot Hospital. 'Look at a young girl these days. She probably starts menstruating at about 12, goes on the pill at about 15 and is on it for years, and then she gets pregnant at 34, 35 or 38 and may have to have fertility drugs to help. She doesn't breast feed for long because she wants to go back to work. Then at 45 she goes on HRT. And during her lifetime she's eaten a low fibre, high carb, high fat diet, she smokes and she doesn't exercise. Look at that same girl 40 years ago and there's no comparison.'

Delightfully, breast cancer is not contagious and massaging, bumping, squeezing or touching breasts does not cause it.

OESTROGENS

Increased oestrogen exposure is implicated in the development of breast cancer.[14] Oestrogen gets a bad rap, but like anything oestrogen has to be found at 'a normal level' within the body. Too little can lead to growth problems, menopausal symptoms, bone loss and can play havoc with the heart and blood vessels. Too much oestrogen exposure over a lifetime may stimulate breast cells to overgrow.

There are two types of oestrogen.
1. **Endogenous oestrogen** is the oestrogen your own body makes.
2. **Exogenous oestrogen** is the oestrogen you are exposed to externally, such as that found in birth control pills (the oral contraceptive pill), hormone replacement therapy (HRT) and xeno-oestrogens. Xeno-oestrogen is a term used to describe a similar substance to oestrogen. It is a by-product of industrial and chemical processes and can interfere with the natural balance of progesterone and oestrogen in the body. Xeno is the Greek word for foreign or strange and xeno-oestrogens are scary for their ability to mimic our own oestrogens.

The body breaks down both of these types of oestrogen and forms either 'good' oestrogen (2-hydroxyestrone) or 'bad' oestrogen (16a-hydroxyestrone). It's quite complicated to explain but to put it simply, bad oestrogen can promote cancer by over stimulating breast cells and activating excessive cell growth and division. Obesity, toxic exposure and alcohol consumption also encourage the body to make bad oestrogen. By encouraging the body to make good oestrogen, or a balanced ratio of good and bad oestrogen, through exercising and cutting back on alcohol and other 'baddies' and increasing the 'goodies', you may lessen the chance of developing breast cancer.

RISK FACTORS

The positive news is that it's possible to look after your breasts, your wellbeing and lessen your risk of manifesting breast cancer. By taking simple measures to lessen these risks you can also improve other health aspects of your life. You can also reduce the possibility of age-related diseases that may include high blood pressure, high cholesterol, obesity, diabetes (Type II, gestational), dementia, arthritis and osteoporosis.[15,16]

The risk factors outlined below shouldn't put you off, make you anxious or stop you considering seeing a health professional for an examination or consultation. Remember, these risk factors are related to the development of breast cancer – not dying. Many of them can be avoided and it's just as important to keep in mind that most women who have these risk factors do not get breast cancer.

At present some of these are considered controversial because many of the studies available conflict with each other.[17] Although there are many risks to consider, some women of increasing age may still develop breast cancer even though there does not appear to be any of the known causative hazards present. There's simply no guarantee we'll all live to 100 years old! There are just some things we cannot control and these include: age, genetics, family history, when we first start menstruating or when menopause occurs. But we can avoid or control the other risks. (See Diagram 2 on page 36.) If you are at all concerned, talk to your health professional sooner rather than later and if possible use healthy strategies to lessen possible threats. Some of this may be scary at first. That's normal, but remember the more you know the less you fear.

What are the known risks for developing breast cancer?

- **Gender:** Breast cancer affects more women than men, however, the outcome is fairly similar in both sexes.
- **Increasing age:** Studies show that as we get older our chance of developing the disease increases, especially after the age of 50. Breast cancer occurs most frequently in women aged between 50 and 65.[18] Although it's rare for women to develop breast cancer before menopause, sadly, it does happen. Breast cancer does not discriminate.
- **Race:** New Zealand European, Maori, Chinese, Indian, other European, and Asian women have a higher breast cancer incidence rate than Pacific women.[19] We don't know if this is because of lack of early detection, however, Pacific and Maori women initially present with more advanced breast disease than these other ethnic groups. Maori women develop more node positive tumours than women from other ethnic groups and Pacific Island women tend to present with larger tumours.[20] Rural Asian women migrating to European countries or adopting the Western diet and way of life also have increased breast cancer risk.
- **History of breast cancer:** If you have already had breast cancer the chance increases of developing it again, either in the same or the other breast.
- **Family history:** The potential to develop breast cancer is increased if a family member has had breast or ovarian cancer. Your family member's age and whether they are first and second generation relatives are taken into account as well.
- **Genetic predisposition:** Health care professionals advise genetic testing and counselling for people who have had other family members present with breast cancer. They look for certain gene mutations, namely BRCA1 on chromosome 17 and BRCA2 on chromosome 13. However, most family history of breast cancer doesn't represent a direct genetic link.

If other family members have mutated genes it does not automatically mean you do. If, however, these genes are found, the risk for developing cancer is increased so you will be closely monitored.

• **Hodgkin's disease:** A cancer that affects the lymph nodes. Those who have had Hodgkin's disease and have undergone radiotherapy to treat it have an increased risk of developing breast cancer.

• **Child bearing:** Having your first child after 35 is thought to have some bearing on breast cancer incidence so, in relation to breast cancer, there's something to be said for becoming a mother at a younger age. Studies on abortion and miscarriage show no increase.

• **Menstruation and menopause:** Women who get their period (menstruate) before the age of 12, and women who experience menopause later (after the age of 55) are believed to be at increased risk because they are exposed to more oestrogen during their lifetime. Oestrogen plays a role in breast cancer because it stimulates the growth of some breast cancers.

• **Hormone therapy:** Oestrogen and progesterone hormone therapy increases our overall exposure to these particular hormones that may play a role in stimulating the growth of abnormal breast cells in some people.

• **Contraceptive hormones (birth control pills):** Is there a link between taking the hormonal contraceptive and breast cancer? Unfortunately there is no straightforward answer as most of the available research is conflicting. Studies have shown that there may be a link between taking the oral contraceptive pill and breast cancer.[21,22] For example, some reports have shown that women who have taken a higher dose oral contraceptive in the past have an increased risk of breast cancer.[23] Other studies and hypotheses show that there is no risk at all, and that the recommended newer low dose oral contraceptives and subdermal implants don't pose any breast cancer risk and are safe to use long-term.[24,25]

• **HRT:** A long-term study showed a large group of women who took hormone replacement therapy (HRT) increased their risk of developing breast cancer.[26] Many women have stopped taking HRT because of this breast cancer risk even though the study showed that the risk is deemed small.[27] These sorts of issues should be discussed with a doctor or health professional you trust as the benefits you gain from HRT may outweigh the risks. If you have particular concerns you could try some of the natural formulations described on page 103.

- **Breast tissue changes:** The changes that occur within breasts are important when it comes to breast cancer risk. Changes in density, the shape, number and size of cells are indicators to our long-term breast health. Breast tissue changes may present as:

  Atypical hyperplasia (AH): A benign (non-cancerous) condition in which cells show abnormal growth in part of the breast. This can occur in the ducts (atypical ductal hyperplasia) or the lobes (atypical lobular hyperplasia).

  Lobular carcinoma *in situ* (LCIS): A benign (non-cancerous) condition that starts in the breast lobules. If you develop LCIS you will be monitored as your breasts, regardless of which side has LCIS, share an increased risk of developing cancer.

  Ductal carcinoma *in situ* (DCIS): A non-invasive cancer in which malignant-appearing cells are contained within the breast duct.

  Age-induced changes: Breast tissue is more glandular when we're young and as we age this tissue is replaced by more fatty tissue and connective fibrous tissue. Women who have particularly fibrous breasts (this can be detected by a mammogram) are at increased risk of breast cancer.

  Benign breast lumps: Women who have experienced benign lumps in their breasts have an increased risk of developing breast cancer.

- **Ignoring breast signs and symptoms:** We've said it before and we must say it again: if you have an abnormal discharge from the breast, nipple retraction, puckering of the breast and/or breast lumps you really should have a check-up. Studies have shown that a longer delay in presenting with breast symptoms is associated with a lower rate of survival from breast cancer.[28]

- **Obesity:** Women who gain excess weight during pregnancy (over 17 kg) increase later breast cancer risk if they don't lose the weight before menopause. (The recommended weight-gain during pregnancy is dependent on your pre-pregnancy weight, but for most women is around 11–16 kg.)[29] And if you are carrying way too much weight after menopause you also have an increased risk. Even though the ovaries are effectively turned off post-menopause, a heavier woman becomes her own oestrogen factory as the body converts the testosterone and androstenedione found in body fat into oestrogen. And because obese women have more body fat they are likely to make more oestrogen than women of a healthy weight. This means they may experience more long-term exposure to oestrogen

and, therefore, have an increased risk of stimulating breast cancer cell growth. Women who tend to store excess fat around the stomach area are more at risk than those who tend to store fat around their thighs and hips.
- **Lack of exercise:** This may contribute to breast cancer. A few hours each week of moderate to vigorous exercise can reduce a woman's exposure to the ovarian hormones that cause breast cancer.[30] And the wonderful by-product of physical activity is that it also reduces obesity (see above), therefore helping lower the risk of breast cancer.
- **Poor nutrition:** There is no doubt we don't see much evidence of vitamin deficiency syndromes, such as scurvy and beriberi, today. However, a less than desirable intake of some vitamins is not uncommon in New Zealand. That's not so good when you know that less than ideal folic acid levels, along with low levels of vitamins B6 and B12, have been found to raise the potential for cardiovascular disease, neural tube defects, and colon and breast cancer.[31,32] Apparently the risk of post-menopausal breast cancer may be increased among women with low intakes of folate if they consume alcohol-containing beverages.[33] And common belief is that a low intake of fresh fruit and/or vegetables and a low intake of wholegrain cereals contributes to greater risk.[34] Two recent studies – one from Cambridge and one from Harvard – found a significant link between animal fat and increased incidence of breast cancer. In the well-known Harvard University Nurses Health Study, a link was shown between premenopausal animal fat intake, mainly red meat and high fat dairy foods, and breast cancer.[35,36]
- **Alcohol:** Sad news for us wine lovers, but drinking more than two standard alcoholic beverages every day is believed to increase breast cancer risk. Of course most of us know red wine consumption at modest levels (read: a glass every second day. One glass is an antioxidant, a bottle is the opposite!!) is known to protect people from diseases, such as heart disease. It's how much you drink and how often that's the key.
- **Smoking:** If you started smoking as a teen and have continued to puff away for at least 20 years your breast cancer risk may be increased.[37] Smoking also increases the risk of breast cancer in post-menopausal women.[38] And just to ensure you know how bad the habit is, it also reduces your survival rate of breast cancer.

2 | ABOUT BREAST CANCER

DIAGRAM ONE

BREAST CANCER RISK FACTORS

- Excessive ionizing radiation exposure
- Environmental factors
- Gene mutations
- Genes (BRCA1, BRCA2)

- Post-menopausal obesity
- Lack of exercise
- Poor nutrition
- Excess alcohol
- Smoking

- Gender
- Age
- Race
- History of cancer
- Family history of breast cancer

- Oral contraceptive use
- HRT use
- Ignoring breast changes and avoiding check-ups

- Breast tissue changes
- Benign breast lumps
- Mammographically dense breasts
- LCIS, DCIS and AH

- Menstruation starting at an early age
- Late menopause
- Not bearing children or bearing children after 35yrs of age

DIAGRAM TWO

HOW TO LESSEN BREAST CANCER RISK

- If you are childbearing age, start your family earlier
  Breast feed

- Eat less animal fat and substitute with essential fatty acids
  Eat more omega 3 and 6 oils

- Avoid having unnecessary x-rays
  Drink fewer than 2 standard serves of alcohol per day
  Exercise

- Take nutritional supplements
  Choose healthy nutrition, fruits and vegetables
  Gain knowledge and empower yourself

- Be a healthy weight
  Be smoke-free
  Have regular breast care check-ups

- (Yet to be proved) Stop taking the oral contraceptive
  Do not take HRT for more than 4 years

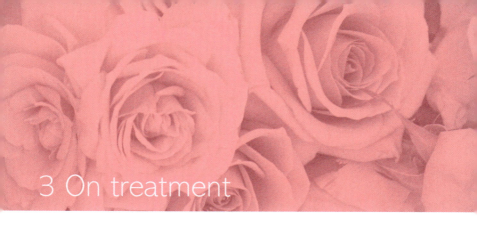

3 On treatment

IF YOU'VE DISCOVERED you have breast cancer you'll be heading into the minefield of treatment. You'll find most breast cancer specialists will explain things clearly and they will help you to feel at ease. But what you're going through is not easy and you'll be looking at all sorts of avenues to possibly help the process along. Many people wonder if the natural way will be of help to them. The good news is that it can be very helpful and can be used in conjunction with traditional (orthodox) medicine. However, you should only take advice on natural therapies from reputable health professionals who specialise in the complex disease that is breast cancer.

Why choose the natural way?

Can you enhance your healing processes after breast cancer surgery, chemotherapy or radiotherapy with natural therapies? Is natural medicine safe? Is it too much effort or too expensive?

These questions are completely valid when it comes to your breasts and your health. Unfortunately there are a lot of myths surrounding natural therapies (also known as complementary alternative medicine or CAM) and they may cause some people to hesitate. A common (yet totally unrealistic) image that springs to mind is someone who looks emaciated, juicing a bag full of organic carrots and munching on celery sticks to 'cure cancer'. Now that's enough to put anyone off! Although juicing is of great benefit, we cannot live on juice alone – more nutrients, knowledge and self-care is needed to help support the body's regeneration and immunity.

CAM, as the name suggests, is complementary to traditional (orthodox) medicine. Herbs, supplements, visualisation and other well-researched natural therapies can be taken or used in conjunction with conventional treatment methods. Nutritional support can help reduce the side effects of medical treatment and enhance healing and wellbeing. There is a lot of scientific research available to prove and validate CAM's worth.

Alternative therapy removes potential energy blocks and allows the body to heal. It involves good old-fashioned common sense and includes lifestyle recommendations, advice on nutrition, supplements and herbs, and even counselling. It can enhance every aspect of your health and life.

The first step is to visit a naturopath, who will look at each individual case and treat it accordingly. What is recommended for one person may not be recommended for another.

In the United States and Europe many orthodox clinics have onsite naturopaths, acupuncturists and nutritionists who offer natural treatment and support alongside the prescribed conventional recommendations and treatments by general practitioners and medical specialists. Ongoing and unfolding research proves the benefits of CAM therapies alongside the conventional. Thousands of successful anecdotal reports have helped pave the way for society to accept natural medicine and support continued research to discover more of the powers of natural medicine.

Unfortunately, there are, and always will be, unqualified, airy-fairy, self-professed natural therapists who offer false hope and expensive, unethical treatments to those in desperate need of help. That's why it's important to empower yourself with as much knowledge as you can about your health and your breasts. We hope that this book helps to steer you in the right direction.

CAM and conventional breast cancer treatment

You may or may not have time to prepare yourself physically and mentally for conventional breast cancer treatment. But, no matter what treatment you're having, there are many ways to enhance your wellbeing before, during and after. Diet, meditation, micronutrients, yoga and herbal medicine are favoured complementary alternative therapies used by breast cancer patients alongside conventional treatment.

Around the world many people are turning to CAM to ensure they have armed themselves with the best nutrition to help counteract the adverse effects of conventional therapies. Internet websites have opened our eyes to what's available. However, there is so much information, it can be quite daunting. Some people find the information too technical, too basic or biased, or favoured towards selling products. And be warned: all too often internet information can be misleading, frightening or full of anecdotal evidence that may not be true.

This can be confusing and most people aren't aware what is safe to take in conjunction with surgery or breast cancer treatment. Surgeons recommend avoiding supplements and CAM because of the lack of concise factual information that is available; they are erring on the side of caution.

ARE THESE SUPPLEMENTS SUGGESTIONS SAFE?

We have only included a few supplements and herbs out of the many that may be available. However, these we have thoroughly researched, sifting through mounds of information, to provide you with supplements and dosages that are safe to take and that work. This is backed by the latest information available.

CAM continues to be investigated by researchers, and the outcomes provide us with good information on means that may improve survival rates, reduce recurrence or relieve associated symptoms of treatment and disease. Further reputable scientific studies on CAM and its effects on breast cancer treatment and care are continually needed.

But first, if you are having treatment, there are some simple practicalities that need to be taken care of.

BEING PRACTICAL AND GETTING FRIENDLY SUPPORT

Tell your friends and family you are having treatment for breast cancer and let them give you moral support during this time. Let good people into your life and heart. Your friends may come up to you and say, 'If there's anything I can do…' Often they want to be helpful, but don't know what to do or say. Allow them time to process their feelings about how it affects them.

You will need a lot of help because it can be very hard doing everything yourself. Friends will offer to do anything they can, so take up the offer. If you like, you can give them jobs to do. Ask them to do things they are capable of or willing to do. If it all seems too much, get someone to draft up a list of jobs you would like done and ask if they can delegate these jobs to your friends and family. Trust us, if they offer to help, they mean it and it gives them an opportunity to do something for you. If the shoe was on the other foot, you'd do it, wouldn't you?

Breast cancer surgery

When a woman is diagnosed with breast cancer it's almost a given she will have to undergo some type of surgery. This may be a lumpectomy, whereby the surgeon only has to remove the part of the breast where the tumour is situated. This is usually followed by radiation therapy. Or a mastectomy may be required where the entire breast needs to be removed. In some cases, the breast and axilla (underarm lymph node or nodes*) may need to be removed also. Sometimes a woman may choose to have a bilateral mastectomy where both breasts are removed so she won't have to worry about breast cancer (although there is a very small possibility – very, very small – of the cancer recurring in the chest wall).

Gone are the days when a breast cancer diagnosis meant radical breast surgery, where a woman would lose her breast and most of her chest wall. The focus these days is on breast conservation surgery and most surgeons are highly skilled. Your surgeon's bedside manner is enormously important. If you don't experience a pleasant, empathetic ear, leave straight away and don't go back. Find someone else, you have quite enough to deal with. Most of the surgeons in this country are delightful but there are always exceptions. Dr Belinda Scott, an Auckland breast surgeon and chair of the New Zealand Breast Cancer Foundation's Medical Committee, says she was inspired to be a breast surgeon by her mentor, Mr John Simpson, a surgeon in Wellington.

'He had the ability to communicate but later I worked with some people who didn't have that knack,' she says. 'I thought it was unfair that women should have someone saying to them "we're just going to take your breast off but you'll be fine darling." I found myself thinking, "hello, there's somebody under there". Women deserve to have good people caring for and nurturing them.'

---

*More and more surgeons are using sentinel node biopsy which removes the first lymph node(s) the cancer may have drained to. This is found by injecting a blue dye into the breast by the tumour before surgery. The dye passes through the system and follows the path to the first draining (sentinel) node(s) the cancer cells are drawn to. If this node proves to be cancerous more nodes may need to be taken. However, if it is clear it may save the need to have further lymph nodes removed which will significantly reduce the incidence of lymphoedema (see page 68). If your surgeon doesn't perform this procedure find someone who does, there is quite a high level of experience and expertise required.

Experts also suggest undergoing surgery in the middle of your menstrual cycle (luteal phase) if you are pre-menopausal. While ongoing studies are underway, some schools of thought believe this may have long-term survival benefits and until definitive evidence is produced it's a choice it wouldn't hurt you to make.[39]

RECONSTRUCTION

Whether or not you choose to have reconstruction is a very personal decision. Some women find the fact that it is possible to undergo reconstruction at the same time as their breast surgery a blessing as it means they never see themselves entirely breastless. Other women prefer not to have reconstruction straight away or ever. And in some cases it is not possible to have breast reconstruction at all. Factors such as stroke, diabetes and heart disease may make the risks too high. Many studies over the past 20 years have shown that breast reconstruction after cancer surgery is safe from a cancer survival point of view.

If you do choose to go ahead with breast reconstruction, and you have realistic expectations, the results can be phenomenal. Breast reconstruction is about creating volume where you've always had a breast and the priority is breast symmetry. The surgeon uses an implant or the body's own tissues to create that volume. An implant can be inserted directly behind the muscle and skin of the chest wall or, in some cases, an expanding technique may be used first. This involves having saline injected into the chest wall over several weeks to 'push' the area out and when it has reached the required size, the implant is inserted. When the body's own tissues are used a section is commonly taken from the tummy (TRAM flap surgery), the back (latissimus dorsi surgery) and occasionally the hips, thighs and buttocks (microvascular surgery).

Most of the time a plastic surgeon will favour using your own tissue, as this technique can have a better result, in terms of looking and feeling like a 'normal' breast. However, performing this type of procedure is difficult and requires a highly trained plastic surgeon. The complicated process involves taking a section of tissue, fat and muscle and moving it elsewhere in the body. During TRAM flap surgery an area from the abdomen is transferred up to the breast area and sewn into place while with latissimus dorsi surgery, back muscle and tissues are moved around to the breast area and sewn into place. In both cases the original arteries and veins are left untouched.

Microvascular surgery, however, takes a section of tissue, fat and muscle from the area, cuts the blood vessels and feeder veins, picks the whole section up and lifts it up to the chest, sews the blood vessels back together, and sews a breast shape into place. Sometimes your other breast may need, or you may want it, to be changed to complement your reconstructed breast. Some women are delighted to have a reduction or uplift on their remaining breast. The surgeon can also mould a nipple for you and an areola and the nipple can be tattooed in the same shade as your other nipple. Tattooing is usually done at a later date when any swelling has subsided. If you do have reconstruction you can expect a hospital stay of about a week and it takes around two to three months to be back to normal. However, most women say they feel pretty good after two to three weeks.

Plastic surgeon Mr Janek Januszkiewicz, who is well known for his breast reconstruction work, feels that from a psychological point of view women do better if reconstruction is done at the time of mastectomy and from his point of view he feels he can achieve a better result. 'Reconstruction has to be right for the woman though,' he says. 'Well-meaning friends may make a woman feel pressured to go ahead and have the surgery, but for some women it may not be the right thing to do. It's a lot of extra surgery and you have to consider whether it is worthwhile for you.' He recently conducted a satisfaction survey of women who had breast cancer surgery and found there was an extremely high level of satisfaction among his reconstruction patients. However, interestingly, women who chose never to have reconstruction were also surveyed and reported good levels of satisfaction with their quality of life.

'The women who were least happy were those on the public system waiting list for reconstruction, they have to wait years which would be extremely difficult,' he says. 'This surgery is about rehabilitating the mind as well as the body. I think reconstruction for the right woman is a fantastic thing. There's a book called *A Woman's Decision* that I think many people would find helpful if they're weighing up the pros and the cons.' (See Further reading to help you through on page 132 for more details.) Reconstruction of any kind is far from a simple technique and it is important to ensure you have a very good plastic surgeon. For recommendations contact the New Zealand Foundation for Cosmetic Plastic Surgery or the New Zealand Medical Council. (See page 131 for contact details.)

How to cope the CAM way with surgery and reconstruction

There are a lot of things you can do to prepare your mind and body for surgery. After all you want to make sure your body has the best chances for recovery and repair. Just being able to do something often makes you feel like you're in control and lessens the worry of surgery.

There are three things you can do primarily to minimise the shock of surgery and enhance your healing.

1. Have the best levels of nutritional micronutrients you can in your body. This will help to negate the effects of medication and anaesthesia, and encourage regeneration of tissues.
2. Organise your personal life to make things easier and reduce stress in the future.
3. Practise a healthy mindset and lifestyle before and after surgery to enhance overall healing rate and wellbeing. This includes reducing or avoiding drinking alcohol, taking recreational drugs and smoking.

NATURAL SUPPLEMENTS TO AID HEALING FOR
SURGERY AND RECONSTRUCTION

Before we go into what herbs and supplements are safe to take and beneficial for healing, we need to know which herbs and supplements to avoid. You don't want to be two weeks down the track and realise you shouldn't have been taking a particular herb or supplement at all.

Herbs and supplements to avoid

While most supplements are generally safe there are a few herbs, nutrients and health oils that should be avoided or used with caution depending on:
- when you have surgery;
- how long your surgery will take;
- what the dose of the supplement is;
- what type of medication you are taking; and
- your health professional's recommendations and monitoring.

Some herbs and supplements can affect medication and prolong bleeding time, which isn't recommended if having surgery, and could raise complications. Use of these substances alone or in combination may increase the anticoagulant effects of each other or prescribed medications. Avoid the following supplements at least two weeks before surgery: St John's wort, ginkgo, ginseng, goldenseal, clove, evening primrose oil, feverfew, fish oil, ginger, garlic, vitamin E, liquorice, red clover, shark cartilage, bovine cartilage, valerian and grapefruit juice.

What to take: two to eight weeks before surgery

Make sure your immune system is strong and healthy before surgery.

You will need to resist the onslaught of opportunistic bacteria that can thrive when your immune system is low. The multi vitamins and minerals contained within immune multis give your body the right nutrients to enhance healing after surgery, to help overcome effects of the general anaesthetic and to assist speed of recovery.

> All the following supplements can be bought at a pharmacy or health store.

Immune Multi Take a low dose immune multi (vitamin, mineral, antioxidants, herbs and nutrients) that is recommended by your natural health practitioner to help your body resist infection, boost immunity and aid healing. Take one daily or as directed. Avoid two weeks prior to surgery. A typical immune multi will include the following.

- **Echinacea** enhances a low immune system by stimulating immune cells to fight off harmful bacteria and viruses. There are no clinical studies documenting adverse reactions using echinacea although most herbalists will not recommend the use of echinacea for transplant patients taking immunosuppressive drugs.[40] Take a low dose of echinacea (250mg–1000mg equivalent of dried rhizome or root of echinacea angustifolia or purpurea).
- **Garlic** has a reputation for thinning the blood, it also acts as an antioxidant and may halt the spread of cancer.[41] It can also kill various bacteria, fungi and viruses.[42] Dose is a key factor when it comes to surgery. Adding garlic to food in small amounts (1–2 cloves a day) is generally considered to be safe, however, you need to be careful when taking large doses of garlic extracts before surgery. Multis normally contain garlic but in quite small doses. Conservatively taking 250mg–500mg equivalent of dried garlic in a multi is fine as long as you stop one to two weeks before surgery to avoid any magnified effects of blood thinning.[43]
- **Mushroom extracts** Aside from the general eating variety we find in the supermarket, certain types of mushrooms found in some immune multis have significant anti-tumour and immune-enhancing properties.[44]
- **Red clover and ginseng** Small amounts of these herbal extracts (<75mg) are used to provide a synergistic effect in immune multis. They both enhance the immune system indirectly. The dose is so low that it does not warrant focus as a dangerous supplement when it comes to

surgery. However, in much higher doses red clover (2g–4g) and ginseng (1.5g–10g) should be avoided prior to surgery.

- **Multi vitamins and minerals** assist the body to fight infections while providing important nutrients for overall health, wound healing and strength of the immune system and body.[45] The normal dose of vitamins and minerals contained in immune multis are generally considered to be quite low doses and safe for surgery. Multis can also include small amounts of amino acids (50mg–100mg) and bioflavonoids (30mg–100mg).
- **Vitamin E** is a powerful antioxidant that is useful for general immune support and healing after surgery, and it may prevent adhesions from internal and external scarring. It may also help the body deal with the adverse effects of drugs. Take 60IU–400IU daily. Avoid two weeks prior to surgery. Although vitamin E is beneficial, caution must be observed when taking vitamin E supplements prior to surgery because of its blood-thinning effects in high doses.[46] Most multis contain small amounts of vitamin E (60IU–150IU). However, some patients take 200IU–400IU daily four to eight weeks before surgery to help prevent adhesions from surgery scarring and promote healing of body tissues. The Food and Nutrition Board of the Institute of Medicine (Washington) established that 1500IU of natural vitamin E (d-alpha-tocopherol) supplements would be the highest dose unlikely to result in haemorrhage in almost all adults.[47] Vitamin E should not be taken one to two weeks prior to surgery to avoid any possibilities of blood-thinning complications leading to haemorrhage.

What to take: one week before surgery
Stop taking all supplements and herbs unless otherwise recommended by a qualified naturopath who is monitoring you and working with your surgeon.

Rescue Remedy This ubiquitous, much-loved security blanket combines five plant essences and can help prepare your body for surgery. It can help remove the feeling of shock or even grief at the thought of surgery. It will also enhance the healing rate of your body and recovery from bruising. It is safe to take before surgery and when you come out of surgery. It will not cause blood thinning or interact with any drugs or cause any complications regarding the surgery. You can add four drops to a bottle of water and sip it throughout the day, or spray it directly into your mouth if you feel stressed, or you can spray it onto your wrists (pulse points).

Homeopathic liquid arnica There is slight confusion about arnica and surgery. Surgeons and doctors need to be aware that arnica that is homeopathically prepared is safe to take before and after surgical operations. Like Rescue Remedy, arnica reduces bruising, helps recovery from anaesthetics and will increase the speed of recovery.

Arnica that is not homoeopathically prepared can be found in anti-bruising creams and as a herbal tincture. It can be toxic internally even at low doses and should not be used by the inexperienced. Arnica that is not homeopathically prepared may also increase blood thinning which is why conventional practitioners who aren't aware of the difference between homeopathic and whole herbs will advise you to avoid arnica at all costs.

Take homeopathic liquid arnica as directed and avoid drinking coffee or eating, using or smelling peppermint or strong aromatics at the same time. These substances can negate the effects of arnica. You can also spray the homeopathic liquid arnica onto your pulse points if you don't want to take it internally under the tongue.

Exercise Gentle stretching and walking can help prepare your body for surgery. Healthy circulation of blood and lymph flow and limber muscles will help your recovery while giving you a chance to relax your mind. Stretch for 20 minutes every day until the day of your surgery.

What to take: after anaesthetic
After awakening from surgery you will feel the effects of the anaesthetic. Feeling groggy, like your head is stuffed with cotton wool, is common. While in hospital avoid any other supplements but continue to take your prescribed medication, homeopathic liquid arnica and Rescue Remedy.
Homeopathic liquid arnica and Rescue Remedy Take your arnica and Rescue Remedy straight away. You should 'come to' immediately and feel much better. Take a minimum of four times daily. Add to your sipping water or spray directly into your mouth or onto pulse points.

What to take: one to four weeks after surgery
Immune multi Continue to take your multi to enhance healing and support your body's immunity. Take one tablet daily or as directed.
Vitamin E Scarring can lead to internal adhesions that can often be

painful as they tear. Take 60IU–400IU daily of vitamin E to enhance healing and prevent adhesions.

Acidophilus is a beneficial bacteria found in digestive flora. If you are taking antibiotics you may need an acidophilus supplement to help repopulate the good bacteria in your gut to ensure digestive health. Take at least 1 billion of acidophilus (and bifidus if combined) daily.

Spirulina is an algae food supplement that is rich in nutrients and protein. It enhances the body's healing rate and aids convalescence. Take 3g daily.

Aloe vera juice assists digestion of nutrients, which is crucial at this time to aid overall healing. Take 50ml before meals to aid digestion and assimilation of nutrients.

Fibre supplements may be necessary when you have undergone surgery and disrupted your eating routine, as you could become constipated. Take fibre supplements as needed and directed.

Scarring After your scars have sealed over (cleanly), apply rosehip oil to the scar and surrounding area to help the scars fade over time. (Do not take internally.)

Exercise Continue to exercise gently. This will induce a deep sleep important for regeneration of cells and energy for the next day. Your energy level will tend to be quite low, which is normal after surgery. Your body has a lot of recovery work to do. Walk for a minimum of 20 minutes every day, unless your health professional advises against it. This will prime your body, circulation and immune system and get it back into optimal condition.

What to do after four weeks?
After four weeks you may be wondering what else you can do. Read and follow the recommendations outlined in risk-reducing strategies for breast cancer on page 81.

Radiotherapy

Radiotherapy, or radiation therapy, has been shown to be very effective in the treatment of breast cancer and can reduce the chance of local recurrence by two-thirds. It acts kind of like a vacuum cleaner after you have a spillage. Say you drop a jar of petals onto the carpet, you pick up the bulk and then suction up the leftover debris. Radiotherapy machines

> A fabulous little exercise to help you get your arm strength back after breast surgery is to walk your fingertips up and down a wall.

are called 'linear accelerators' which shoot beams at a target area and the suction analogy above equates to the radiotherapy beams which 'hoover' up any leftover cancer cells. A course of radiotherapy is typically given for five minutes each day, five days per week for five weeks. Usually it takes place about six weeks after surgery when any scarring should have healed. It is given in small doses frequently as this helps protect the normal tissues in the area being treated. You may undergo chemotherapy before radiotherapy or concurrently (but this occurs less frequently), it depends on the type of chemotherapy you're having. On the first visit for planning the radiation oncologist will use tiny dot tattoos to delineate the area to be treated. (These are usually permanent but you can ask about having them removed after treatment, laser removal should be able to take care of this.) This shows clearly where to aim the photon beams and means the exact same area is treated every day. You will lie on the linear accelerator with your arm raised over your head. This treatment can leave you feeling very tired and it can have a sunburn-like effect on the area that has been radiated. If that happens, a lot of women swear by rubbing pure aloe vera (from the broken leaf) or dabbing aloe vera juice on the area.

There is big movement in this area of breast cancer radiation treatment with perhaps the biggest news being intraoperative radiotherapy. Working on the premise that recurrences usually occur in the original area of the cancer, this area is radiated while the person is still on the operating table. Then there is brachytherapy and MammoSite, which complete radiotherapy treatment within one week. These treatments deliver radiation to the space left in the breast after a tumour has been removed. With MammoSite a single balloon catheter is inserted through a small incision in the breast with its end finishing outside the breast. The balloon is inflated with saline and twice a day for five days you would visit the clinic and be attached to a computer-controlled machine by the piece of the catheter that is outside the breast. This enables delivery of a radioactive seed into the balloon where it emits radiation. After treatment the radioactive seed is removed and you can return home or to work. Brachytherapy is similar, however, several catheters are used instead of the balloon catheter. The fabulous thing about it is that scarring is minimal and it doesn't disrupt your life as traditional radiotherapy can do. The success rates with this treatment in America are huge. Unfortunately, at the time of writing, neither of these techniques is available in New Zealand.

3 | ON TREATMENT

WHAT TO TAKE TO HELP YOU THROUGH RADIATION TREATMENT

Nutritional and naturopathic support during radiation may offer the benefits of reduced side effects, increased tumour cell eradication and higher treatment tolerance.

Omega 3 fish oil has a beneficial effect on cancer patients and appears to increase the effect of radiation, resulting in eradication of a larger number of cancerous cells.[48] Take 3g daily for a minimum of six weeks.

Vitamin B3 (niacin) should always be considered as part of a broad spectrum nutritional supplementation programme. Literature supports the suggestion that niacin supplementation normalises cancer cells and reduces the side effects of radiation, and offers protection against the development of further cancer.[49,50] Take 30mg–60mg daily.

> You are asked not to use deodorant when having radiotherapy, which can be a bit daunting, particularly if you're having treatment in high summer. Try Naturally Fresh, an alternative created especially for cancer patients going through radiation and medical oncology (phone 0800 844 769). It's also a good idea to invest in some unscented soap for the shower.

Magnesium deficiency has been observed with radiation therapy.[51] It has been suggested that besides causing cancer and depleting the body's nutrition stores, magnesium deficiency can lead to a wide range of symptoms and diseases and is crucial for cellular function.[52,53] Take 100mg–2g every eight hours with food to prevent low levels of magnesium.

Selenium New Zealand soil is almost depleted of selenium. This means that we are not getting enough of it in our diets so we must consider supplementation. Selenium is protective against the ongoing side effects of radiation and has shown radioprotective effects in vitro and vivo.[54] Take 200mcg of L-selenomethionine daily.

Radium nosode You will need to see a classical homeopath to obtain a radium nosode. It is a homeopathically prepared remedy that helps negate the side effects of radiation and provides general support for your body's recovery.[55] Take 5–10 drops three times daily.

Aloe vera juice and digestive enzymes help to increase digestive juices thus breaking down foods properly. This can help relieve indigestion and poor assimilation of nutrients. You need to think about nutrition to enhance your recovery rate. Digestive enzyme formulas may include bromelain, papain, lactase, cellulose, phytase, pepsin, peptidase, lipase and betaine. Take digestive enzyme formulas as directed. Take 50ml of aloe vera juice before meals daily.

For radiation burns Aloe vera jelly can be applied to the burn area to relieve pain and aid deep healing of tissues. Aloe vera has a reputation for enhancing skin healing nine times faster than the normal rate. Alan Black™ Animal jelly or Alan Black™ Pure jelly is an excellent brand of medically manufactured and prepared aloe vera gel. Apply as often as needed.

> SUPPLEMENT SUMMARY
> **Vitamin B3 (Niacin)** Take 30mg–60mg daily with food.
> **Magnesium** Take 100mg–2g every 8 hours with food.
> **Selenium** Take 200mcg of L-selenomethionine daily.
> **Aloe vera juice** and **digestive enzymes** Take a digestive enzyme formula as directed. Take 50ml of aloe vera juice before meals daily.

Chemotherapy

Chemotherapy uses anticancer drugs to stop cancer cells dividing, multiplying and surviving. There are so many scary stories about chemotherapy that the very mention of the word is enough to make you feel ill. Being faced with undergoing the treatment is daunting so don't be too hard on yourself if you're feeling fearful at the prospect. While experts say they've come a long way and the treatment is nowhere near as gruelling as it once was, it can still cause hair loss, nausea and infertility. Unfortunately, as of this writing, it's often the best weapon we've got. In future years people will probably look back in the history books and think what a barbaric treatment it was. You see, chemotherapy cannot be specifically targeted to cancer cells (although work is being done on this as we speak). It attacks actively growing cells in the body, both good and bad, and we hope it kills the villain and his gang (cancer cells). In the process though, normal innocent cells get killed as well. The good news is that most of the good guys can grow back. At the moment the chemotherapy formula given is based on the height and weight of the patient but this could change very soon. A promising new genetic profiling test has been shown to accurately predict which breast cancer patients will benefit from chemotherapy and which will not. That's enormously good news because it means that, potentially, some women will be able to safely skip this part of treatment.

On the positive side, chemotherapy is a powerful aid in the treatment of breast cancer and has been shown to improve survival. It works by using a combination of drugs that are given intravenously or via a pill. They make their way through the entire system (this is called systemic treatment) and interfere with the normal process of cell division, ultimately killing cells. You need an expert medical oncologist when you're being treated as its pretty potent stuff. Treatment is given in cycles (usually three or four weeks) which allows a recovery period for the good guy cells. This also takes into account that the cancer cells aren't all active at the same time so it means a continuous attack is being mounted on them as they retreat and come forth. You may be given blood tests between treatments to ensure your blood count is doing OK; this depends on what part of the body is being treated. If your red blood cell count is down you could be tired and on the road to anaemia and if your white blood cell count is down you could be vulnerable to infection. This is where a strong immune system comes in. Part of the immune system's job is to recognise and eliminate cancerous and precancerous cells from the body. Once chemotherapy has zapped enough cancer cells the immune system should be able to stand on its own two feet and do the job it was designed to do. However, during chemotherapy treatment your immunity will probably experience a few knocks, so treat yourself well. Chemotherapy treatment usually lasts three to six months and your body will most likely take that time again to recover.

AC AND CMF

AC (Adriamycin, Cyclophosphamide) and CMF (Cyclophosphamide, Methotrexate, Fluorouracil) are the most common chemotherapies in New Zealand but sometimes newer drugs may be added or used instead.

With AC chemotherapy four injections of AC are given every three weeks over three months. Unfortunately hair loss is a very common side effect with this treatment but your fertility may be retained – something to be considered seriously if you're pre-menopausal. (The risk of infertility is dependent on how old you are when you receive treatment – the older you are the greater your chances of becoming infertile.)

CMF usually involves 12 injections over six months in addition to two weeks of daily tablet taking every four weeks. Injections are given at the beginning and in the middle of treatment. Even though not everyone loses their hair with this course of treatment, it does raise the odds of becoming infertile.

The bad news for both treatments, and there's no way of sugar coating this, is that you could experience nausea, vomiting, diarrhoea or constipation, mouth sores, loss of periods for a time, loss of hair on the scalp and also eyelashes and eyebrows, fuzzy thinking (chemo brain) and fatigue. You may also go into premature menopause.

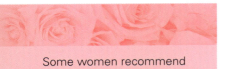

Some women recommend having chemotherapy on a full stomach, eating crystallized ginger, oatmeal, yoghurt, chicken soup, cream crackers or drinking flat cola, chocolate milkshakes or green tea.

One side effect of chemotherapy that's often not talked about is taste. After treatment, people will often associate the food they ate during treatment with feeling nauseous and the change in taste that the treatment can bring on. Coffee and meat can take on a bitter metallic taste. Some people suggest eating meat cold or at room temperature and many women have suggested avoiding your favourite foods during treatment. It is not uncommon to experience food cravings or increased appetite either.

A couple of suggestions to get rid of the taste are to try rinsing with a mix of one teaspoon of baking soda in a cup of water before or between meals and try mint lollies or frequent brushing.[56] 'Many women can tolerate treatment well and are able to work and continue to run a house and look after children,' says Dr Nicole McCarthy. 'You are not sick in bed the whole time you are being treated and you will recover. This doesn't happen immediately, it can take months for energy levels to come back to what they were, but please be assured that eventually they will.'

The other downside to chemotherapy treatment is the risk of gaining weight. The longer your treatment is for, the more likely it is you will experience weight gain. Some of the reasons for this are that you will find you probably exercise less, you may eat more to comfort yourself or to try to combat nausea, and some of the associated drugs can increase your appetite. And if you do go into chemo-induced menopause you may struggle with the associated weight gain.

And then there's 'chemo brain'. Chemo brain is very real. It can manifest in a shorter attention span, less mental flexibility, loss of memory and a slowing in the processing of information. It can be frustrating because you'll forget simple things like people's names. The good news is that you will regain your former alertness.

LOOKING AFTER YOURSELF DURING CHEMOTHERAPY

Supplements can be helpful during chemotherapy. The main aim of natural supplementation is to help replace the nutrients lost through chemotherapy, reduce the adverse effects of chemotherapy and enhance recovery and quality of life.[57,58]

Vitamin B3 (niacin) has offered a small amount of relief from signs and symptoms for patients undergoing chemotherapy.[59] Cancer patients can become niacin deficient after chemotherapy. Niacin is important for healthy cell (DNA) repair, to reduce free radical toxicity, protect bone marrow from chemotherapy damage and reduce further possible cancer development including secondary tumours.[60,61,62] Take 30mg–60mg daily.[63]

Vitamin C deficiencies can lead to cell damage and thus cancer, and may increase the adverse side effects of chemotherapy.[64,65] Although there needs to be more studies for breast cancer chemotherapy treatment and supportive effects of vitamin C supplementation, some studies already completed have proved promising for the use of vitamin C with chemotherapy. Children undergoing chemotherapy for leukaemia showed that supplementing with antioxidants including vitamin C for six months resulted in fewer days spent in hospital and less toxicity from chemotherapy.[66]

Other studies show vitamin C may even enhance the effect of the chemotherapy drug 5-Fluorouracil against cancer cells and chemo-resistant cell lines.[67]

The effectiveness of chemotherapy treatment against ovarian cancer is thought to be enhanced when used in combination with supportive supplementation of vitamins C and E, beta carotene and Coenzyme Q10.[68] Take 1000mg–2000mg of Ester C® vitamin C daily in divided doses with food.

Vitamin E supports the immune system during chemotherapy.[69] One study suggests that vitamin E can be safely taken with the chemotherapy drug Cisplantin, possibly decreasing damage to peripheral nerves.[70] Take 400IU–600IU daily.

Magnesium deficiency is a common side effect of the chemotherapy drug Cisplantin and can affect up to 90 per cent of patients.[71,72] It has been suggested that magnesium deficiency can lead to a wide range of symptoms and diseases. Magnesium is crucial for cellular function, reducing nerve pain, muscle cramps, migraines and the side effects of methotrexate-induced burning pain on the soles of feet and palms of hands.[73,74,75] Magnesium is safe to take with Cisplantin.[76] At present the magnesium dose regarding chemotherapy has not been properly reviewed, however, 100mg is possibly enough to help reduce pain and 2g every eight hours during Cisplantin therapy is the minimum to prevent magnesium deficiency. Take 100mg–2g every eight hours with food.

Selenium is a mineral that is severely depleted in New Zealand soil. Selenium is essential to make antioxidant scavenging enzymes within the body to help prevent cancer and ensure recovery from chemotherapy. Epidemiological studies and trials support the role of selenium as a potent cancer chemopreventive agent because deficiencies in it can lead to cell mutation and breakages.[77,78] It's important for New Zealanders to supplement with selenium to prevent deficiency. A selenium and vitamin E study (SELECT) proposes 200mcg daily of L-selenomethionine for chemoprotection.[79]

Zinc can assist compromised immunity, poor appetite, mental fatigue, poor wound healing, taste and smell problems, which unfortunately can often occur as a side effect of chemotherapy. Methotrexate chemotherapy can cause the digestive tract to become inflamed leading to digestive discomfort, compromised immunity and food sensitivities. Zinc and selenium can reduce these side effects while enhancing the immune system function, healing and recovery.[80] Chemotherapy patients also have a better chance of remission if they have high levels of zinc stores in the body.[81] Look at your nails. Do they have tiny white marks (spots) within the finger nail? Look at your tongue. Do you see any raised single lumps? If you do, you could be zinc deficient now. Take 30mg daily with food.

Beta 1.3 Glucan is a fibre compound that can be derived from the cell walls of yeast. By attaching to immune cell receptors (macrophages) it stimulates an immune response to recognise and destroy mutated cancer cells. Cyclophosphamide chemotherapy used in combination with beta 1.3 glucan has been shown to inhibit more cancer cells, reducing cancer metastasis, than when used on its own.[82,83] It is

3 | ON TREATMENT

thought to have positive effects on boosting interferon and bone marrow. Take 200mg–600mg daily.

Aloe vera juice and digestive enzymes help to increase digestive juices, thus breaking down foods properly. This can help relieve indigestion and poor assimilation of nutrients. You need to think about nutrition to enhance your recovery rate. Digestive enzyme formulas may include bromelain, papain, lactase, cellulose, phytase, pepsin, peptidase, lipase and betaine. Take a digestive enzyme formula as directed. Take 50ml of aloe vera juice before meals daily.

N.B. Not all of the chemotherapy drugs mentioned here are commonly used and it's important to note that it would be rare that any of them would be used on their own.

> SUPPLEMENT SUMMARY
> **Vitamin B3 (niacin)** Take 30mg–60mg daily with food.
> **Vitamin C** Take 1000mg–2000mg of Ester C® vitamin C daily in divided doses with food.
> **Vitamin E** Take 400IU–600IU daily.
> **Magnesium** Take 100mg–2g every 8 hours with food.
> **Selenium** Take 200mcg of L-selenomethionine daily.
> **Zinc** Take 30mg daily.
> **Beta 1.3 Glucan** Take 200mg–600mg daily.
> **Digestive enzymes** Take as directed.
> **Aloe vera juice** Take 50ml before meals daily.

Other nutritional support to consider during chemotherapy includes:[84]

- **Protein powders** to prevent protein malnutrition. Take 30g three times daily. See a nutritionist or naturopath for product recommendation.
- **Glutamine** to help prevent hair loss, immune suppression and inflammation of the digestive system. Take 100mg–250mg daily.
- **Glutathione** to protect your tissues and enhance drug efficacy while reducing toxicity associated with chemotherapy. Glutathione is a powerful antioxidant. Take 2g daily.
- **Prebiotic formulas** to correct and maintain normal beneficial gut flora of the digestive tract. Bacteria, fungi, viruses and parasites can thrive when the immune system is lowered or compromised with any immunosuppressant therapy. Take as directed.

Hormonal treatments

About 60 per cent of breast cancers require the female hormones oestrogen or progesterone to grow. These are known as ER-positive (oestrogen) or PR-positive (progesterone) and are termed 'hormone sensitive' cancers. Hormonal therapies aim to shut down the ovaries and block the supply of these hormones that allow a tumour to flourish. The best known of these treatments is Tamoxifen, which has been around since the 1970s. It has been gold standard for this type of treatment for a long time, however, newer therapies are contesting its superiority. Aromatase inhibitors came to the fore in the 1990s when it was found they could reduce oestrogen levels in the blood. However, they were found to only be useful in post-menopausal women.

A recent study has found an aromatase inhibitor – Anastrozole (Arimidex) – to be extremely effective in the treatment of hormone sensitive cancers in post-menopausal women. The study, known as the ATAC trial, tested three groups of women. One group were given Tamoxifen, one group were given Anastrozole and the third group were given a combination of the two. The study found the women who were given Anastrozole had less recurrence or spread of their cancer over the other groups. It also showed a lower incidence in the cancer spreading to the other breast.[85] Confused? Basically, the difference between a treatment such as Tamoxifen and aromatase inhibitors, such as Anastrozole, is that aromatase inhibitors block the production of oestrogen in post-menopausal women and Tamoxifen blocks the effects of oestrogen at the tumour cell.

NEW THERAPIES

Herceptin is another treatment that should be mentioned here. It is an antibody that is given to women with advanced HER2 positive cancers and has proven to be very effective in the 30 per cent of breast cancers that fall into this category. Experts feel the discovery of Herceptin heralds a whole new wave of anticancer treatments. It is likely that Herceptin will be included in the treatment for women with early stage HER2 positive breast cancer in the future – the results of clinical trials are pending. Recently worldwide trials involving more than 5000 women (including 31 New Zealanders) have shown that when Herceptin is used with chemotherapy after surgery, the chance of the cancer recurring more than halves.

3 | ON TREATMENT

There are also trials underway or planned to test whether some or all of these treatments may help prevent breast cancer. These treatments depend on a number of variances and you can only make an informed decision by discussing these with your medical oncologist. However, the positive news you can pick up from this abbreviated information on hormonal therapies is that more discoveries, and rather powerful ones at that, are being made every day.

SIDE EFFECTS

Tamoxifen side effects can include: hot flushes, vaginal discharge or irritation, irregular periods, nausea, dizziness and weight gain (may be temporary).

Anastrozole left more women feeling achy in their muscles and joints compared with Tamoxifen, however, fewer women experienced hot flushes, blood clots, vaginal bleeding or endometrial cancer. There is also an increased risk of osteoporosis compared with Tamoxifen, which actually protects your bones.

SUPPLEMENTS

Citrus bioflavonoids People should avoid taking Tamoxifen with citrus bioflavonoid supplements also known as quercitin, rutin and tangeretin. Preliminary research in animals found that the citrus flavonoid tangeretin (found primarily in the peel of citrus fruits) interferes with the ability of Tamoxifen to inhibit tumor growth. Although the evidence is far from conclusive, people taking Tamoxifen should probably avoid citrus bioflavonoid supplements, and possibly beverages and foods to which citrus peel oils have been added.[86] Small amounts found in fruits and multis are probably too small to worry about but if you are concerned you should tell your doctor or specialist so they can take this into consideration as they monitor the effects of your medication.

Evening primrose and borage oils contain gamma-linolenic acid (GLA). GLA may enhance the therapeutic effects of Tamoxifen. A small group of breast cancer patients took 2.8g of oral GLA per day in addition to Tamoxifen in a preliminary trial.[87] Another group of breast cancer patients took Tamoxifen alone. Those taking the GLA–Tamoxifen combination appeared to have a better clinical response than did those taking Tamoxifen alone. However, the results of this preliminary research are far from conclusive and need to be confirmed in a larger, more definitive trial.

Tocotrienols are compounds similar to vitamin E that are found in palm oil. Studies have shown that tocotrienols enhance the effects of Tamoxifen although, at this time, more controlled studies are needed to support this theory.[88]

What to do when treatment is over

Whew, that's over! What a mission. You'll no doubt be feeling exhausted and wrung out. But if you want to keep up your natural health supplements, follow the risk-reducing strategies for breast cancer on page 81. Preliminary tests show that supplementing with vitamins A (beta carotene), C and E, selenium, secondary vitamins and minerals, omega 3 and 6 essential fatty acids and Coenzyme Q10 could help improve the outcome of breast cancer, which is promising. Twenty to thirty per cent of women in a group of 32 who had breast cancer found that when they took these supplements they felt their quality of life improved.[89]

Coenzyme Q10 may be important for protection against breast cancer and supportive as a supplement with conventional treatment of breast cancer.[90] As we age or take certain cholesterol or blood pressure medication, CoQ10 becomes depleted, creating deficiencies. Because of CoQ10's role in immunity and involvement in healthy DNA synthesis, it has been investigated in the role of breast cancer therapy support. Studies have so far been very promising. In addition to the above study, two women with metastatic breast cancer received 390mg of CoQ10 for over 11 months. In one patient, the shadows (metastases) in her liver disappeared and in the other patient, no signs of pleural cancer were present after six months.[91,92]

4 Exploring the side effects of having breast cancer

Psyche

YOUR PSYCHE will go through an enormous amount of emotive cycling during this period of your life. You are faced with a potentially (please note the word *potentially*) life-threatening illness and you are going to come up against a whole raft of issues such as betrayal and anger, feelings of fear, grief and bereavement, relationship, body image and femininity issues.

There is an unspoken rule in our society that we should be smiling and laughing as often as possible and this includes during hard times. Some tears and down-times are tolerated by others, but not too many. We're supposed to 'think positive'. But do you know what? Phooey to that. There are some curveballs that life throws at you where you just can't think positive all of the time and a cancer diagnosis is one of them. So give yourself permission to feel whatever you feel and don't worry about anybody else. You are the important one here.

One of the givens of going through any extraordinarily challenging life situation is that you'll find everybody is there for you during the initial crisis. However, as time goes on, and this is something inherent to human nature, some people will fade away. But whatever happens you mustn't feel obliged to smile through your tears. Some people just aren't strong enough to cope with other people's trauma. And in some instances, they quite simply don't understand. The old saying 'walk a mile in someone's shoes' comes into play here. With some people it's simply not in their nature to be supportive in crises, while others have no way of knowing what a situation as enormous as the one you're dealing with feels like.

If your support systems – friends, families and partners – aren't strong, it will be especially hard for you. These are the bonds that create an ability to weather any storm and these hard times are where counselling comes in. The counsellors at the Cancer Society are all professionally trained and specialise in dealing with cancer. What's more, an appointment with them is free and you can go as often as necessary, at the beginning of your breast cancer or three to six months down the track, whenever suits you. 'There still seems to be a stigma towards counselling in our society, and this prevents people getting the support they need,' says Judy Forsythe, who oversees the counselling services at the Auckland Cancer Society. 'Everyone is an individual in how they respond both physically and psychologically to their breast cancer diagnosis. We're there to help people process what they're going through and we specialise in this area.' The counselling division of the Cancer Society has only been going for five years which shows us just how far we've come in terms of recognition of the psychological impacts of the illness.

Speaking to someone who has specialist cancer counselling experience is invaluable and studies show that women who choose to have counselling cope better with their illness than those who don't. 'People are given a great deal of help with their physical healing after surgery, chemotherapy and radiotherapy, but often worry that they might be judged or labelled if they seek the support of a professional counsellor,' says Judy. 'Emotional and psychological healing is just as important if people are to make a complete recovery from an episode of cancer, and I would urge anyone who is struggling to "get back to normal", or feeling pressurised to cope as well as they did prior to their diagnosis, to get in touch with us. We can help with many issues and difficulties that are part of a very normal process of accommodation to the changes brought about by having a diagnosis of breast cancer.' (We ask you to have a talk with the counsellors if you feel the need also – they're lovely people. Contact your local Cancer Society listed in the back of this book.)

Psychiatrist David Spiegel, in his book *Living Beyond Limits*, suggests patients should feel free to talk about whatever concerns them, from fear of losing their breast to fear of dying. In a landmark study Dr Spiegel found that women with breast cancer who received standard medical care and met with a weekly support group experienced less depression, anxiety and pain than women who received no social support.[93]

We must again reiterate that you needn't fall prey to the pressure to be upbeat and/or buy into the common millennium catchphrase, 'think positive and everything will be fine'. If all you want to do is roll up into a ball and cry, do it. But do bear in mind that if you continue feeling like this 24 hours a day for a period of time, it's probably not such a good thing (see Depression on page 62). A 1999 study published in *The Lancet* found that a 'fighting spirit' did not appear to affect healing. 'It is important to say that many women with breast cancer will feel low and helpless from time to time. This might be normal given what they are coping with. Patients who find it difficult to maintain a positive fighting spirit all the time should be relieved of the worry and guilt that they might be causing their cancer to progress. We can reassure them that this is not so,' say the authors of the study.[94]

There are many support groups for women (and men) going through breast cancer and any one of the organisations listed in the resources at the back of this book may help you. Or you may find comfort in prayer, meditation, yoga, creative visualisation, singing, dancing, art, crafts or helping others. In the end everyone will deal with cancer differently. It is a huge burden to shoulder and you must give yourself permission to realise that, be kind to yourself and help yourself (and accept help from others) in any way you can.

What do I tell the children?

If you have dependent children a breast cancer diagnosis is a biggie to explain. Of course it depends on what age they are as to what you tell them and when. But do tell them. A child will often sense something is wrong and if you say nothing at all they may come up with all sorts of situations in their own minds. It is best to sit them down and explain your illness straight away, that way you can outline the process to them; what cancer is, what happens during treatment, why you feel ill, why you've lost your hair (if you do), why you're sad, etc. All of these things are important and, as much as you are on a learning curve, so are your children.

> **OUR ADVICE**
>
> Give yourself permission to have down days, talk about what you are feeling with someone else – this may be a friend, a partner, someone who is going through the same thing or a counsellor, whoever you feel comfortable talking to. Find something you enjoy doing that distracts you from what you're going through. One woman we know concentrated on painting beautiful pieces of art, another took up swimming, another took up writing a journal and yet another redecorated her house. Whatever works for you.

Again the Cancer Society counsellors can help out here and will work together with you and the children or work with you on your own, specifically guiding you on how to find the right words. 'Be honest, reliable and try to ensure what you're telling your children is age-appropriate,' says Judy. 'At the same time it's important to answer questions honestly.'

If your children are under five they fear separation, strangers and being left alone, so they will need the reassurance of knowing you are coming home from hospital soon and that they have done nothing to cause your illness. Children from six to 11 will worry and need support and reassurance. Teenagers, as always, are a difficult age group. They may experience all sorts of confusion with your illness. Try to encourage them to talk about your illness with someone they feel comfortable with, reassure them and try not to burden them with too many extra chores that you are unable to do. Of course they should pull their weight and they may feel better for being able to help, but it's a fine line between feeling valued and feeling put-upon. They still need guidance and support.[95]

Depression

The odds of becoming depressed after the diagnosis and/or experience of breast cancer are quite high. Studies show 10–17 per cent of women experience major depression three months after diagnosis. After 12–24 months those statistics change to 5–20 per cent.[96] If you do suffer from the blues, don't whatever you do beat yourself up about it. You're only human and you've been hit by one of the most stressful situations that can befall a person. On top of having breast cancer you may be alone, your partner may not understand or talk about the disease, you may have to give up your job and be struggling financially or you may be juggling a job, home and family. If you feel consistently hopeless or helpless and find the feeling of joy has become elusive, if you can only see the negative, if you can't drag yourself out of bed, if you're constantly weeping, if you're missing appointments and medication, not exercising or eating and avoiding people, chances are you're depressed. And you need help now! Depression is quite simply awful. So is having cancer. Dealing with a combination of the two is an extreme challenge. Doctors are all too quick to prescribe a bottle of pills to make it go away but some of the other avenues we discuss later in the book also have a very good success rate. It's ironic that cancer and depression can bring on the same symptoms:

loss of appetite, weight changes, trouble sleeping and fatigue.

Try to keep your mind on positive activities and watch out for triggers that make your depression worse or increase the possibility of a relapse. Write notes and possible triggers in a daily diary to help identify these factors. Stimulants such as caffeine, cigarettes, drugs and alcohol can often make depression worse as it can put extra stress on your adrenal glands and deplete protective nutrients. We've all learned to have coping mechanisms and if any of these are yours, it's going to be a bit difficult to just cut them out. Maybe you could start by cutting down a little every day to help wean yourself off. Learn how to relax by trying yoga, gentle exercise, receiving a massage or learning meditation or breathing techniques. And remember to get plenty of restful sleep. Make sure the room is completely dark to help ensure a deep slumber.

GOOD MOOD FOODS AND SUPPLEMENTS

Yes, there is such a thing as feel-good food! Complex carbohydrates create serotonin, which is an important mood brain-chemical that normally floods the brain cells to make you feel happy. When it's not released in sufficient quantities depression can strike. Small-portioned complex carbohydrate meals throughout the day can increase the production of serotonin and emotional energy.

Complex carbohydrates, such as legumes, whole-grain breads, pasta and cereals, starchy vegetables, such as potatoes, and carrots are wonderful ingredients for your body when it comes to making serotonin.

The key is to combine protein with all your complex carbohydrate meals. Protein is broken down into an amino acid called tryptophan, a precursor ingredient to 5-hydroxytryptophan (5HTP) and serotonin. (Yes, gobbledygook science, but that's how it works.) For example, tuna and caper pasta with herbed tomato sauce is a satisfying low calorie meal that can supply your protein, carbohydrate and omega 3 needs.

Why omega 3? Omega 3 is a good fat that is found in plants, seafood and fish, such as tuna and salmon. If you don't get enough omega 3 in your diet, you can get moody and depressed. Fish oil and flax seed oil supplements relieve feelings of irritation, put a halt to spontaneous tears and, as a bonus, nourish hair, skin and nails.

5HTP can help normalise low serotonin levels. The health supplement ingredient 5HTP is naturally sourced from the African griffonia plant. It really helps to lift your spirits but can take a week or two to really kick in.

Take 150mg–300mg daily and then a maintenance amount of 50mg daily when you feel the blues begin to dissipate.

Besides 5HTP other mood-altering supplements include B complex multis, iron, calcium, magnesium and the herbs St John's wort, ginseng, passionflower and Californian poppy.

Nutritional supplements can aid the adrenal glands and immune system and also help to relieve depression. Look for a B complex multi with extra B5 and herbs for healthy adrenal function. It normally takes four days to a week to feel like it is starting to work.

Bach™ Flower remedies such as elm, gorse, cherry plum and Rescue Remedy can help with the emotional symptoms of depression. Feelings of being overwhelmed, not being able to see the light at the end of the tunnel, shock, guilt, panic and fear can be helped with Bach™ Flowers. A naturopath can mix your specific remedy. These really do work. Take 4 drops minimum 4 times daily or if needed take 4 drops every five minutes.

Tissue Salt Kali Phos, a homeopathic mineral, is excellent for nerves and depression, and can work very quickly without being contraindicated with other medication. Take 1 tablet minimum 4 times daily or if needed take 1 tablet every five minutes.

Fatigue

They say the fatigue that commonly accompanies treatment for breast cancer is indescribable. Perhaps most frustrating is that you look fine but each day your body feels like it doesn't want to move. Couple this with loss of interest in people and activities and you'll find it hard to get out of bed.

There is no telling when fatigue might hit – once again it's different for everybody. Some people find it hardest during treatment and some don't experience it until it's all over. And there's no way of knowing how long this washed-out feeling will last. Some say it can take six to eight months depending on the duration of your treatment. Others say it may go on for years. Fatigue can also be a symptom of depression or it can make you vulnerable to depression.

One woman we know ensured she walked every day and firmly believes this is why she didn't experience the crushing fatigue that so many people describe. If you don't feel up to exercise try doing things in the parts of the day where you have slightly more energy. Or just go with it if you can.

Read, listen to music and spend time with others who don't put excessive expectations on you. There are so many people out there who are quick to say, 'Oh, aren't you over that by now?' Don't let them into your space, instead surround yourself with people who will help you laugh and respect where you're at. And if you're not lucky enough to be able to have someone to clean for you then you might have to let go of any overzealous cleaning habits you have. It's funny how sometimes the perfect house with floors-you-can-eat-off loses its importance. Most of the medics say your energy should come back very slowly. Expect to have good days and bad days. This is one occasion where you may have to live moment by moment.

REMEDIES

Spirulina is one of the best remedies for fatigue. It is chemoprotective, radioprotective and safe to take to help your body recover after surgery. Mix 1 tsp of spirulina with milk (rice, soy, cow's) or fruit juice and drink. If you don't feel up to making a smoothie, spirulina comes in tablets too. You need 3g three times daily to help put nutrition back into your body. Think about seeing a naturopath so they can make a herbal formula and a nutrition plan specifically for you.

Grief

Grief is one of the hallmarks of any catastrophic life event and in order to deal with it you need to understand it. There is a well-respected grief curve created by Granger Westberg author of *Good Grief*.[97] It works in steps beginning from the time when you fall over the edge and go into grief. You need sensitive and supportive people around you while you come to terms with what you are facing. The steps of Westberg's curve go like this (bear in mind the order might be different for you). He says it is normal for it to take 18 to 24 months to move through the process.

1. Shock and denial – you may feel numb and dazed.
2. Express feelings – you may vacillate between crying, screaming and sobbing in powerful outbursts.
3. Body reactions – sleeping, eating, breathing may all be disrupted and you are consumed by your emotions.
4. Depression and panic – you may feel hopeless and like the darkness will never end.
5. Guilt – blaming yourself. If only you'd eaten differently, etc.
6. Anger – why me? Your anger may feel irrational.

7. Idealisation – you feel that the past was perfect and things will never be any good again.

8. Realisation – acceptance begins and you begin to come to terms with where you are at.

9. New patterns – you start to make the changes that are necessary to accommodate the ways in which your life may have changed. You may at this point make major changes with where you live, work and in your relationships.

10. Living with the loss – you've walked a very trying journey but have come to re-evaluate your life. You will never forget what you've experienced but you've accepted it and are back on an even keel.

> ## REMEDIES
>
> The Bach™ Flower essence Rescue Remedy is wonderful for grief, which at times feels all-consuming and overwhelming, leaving you feeling numb and vulnerable. Take two sprays four times a day or use as needed.

Guilt

'Regarding this let me be absolutely clear – you did not cause your breast cancer,' says Dr John Link in *Take Charge of Your Breast Cancer*.[98] Hear! hear! Many people go through a period of time when they feel that something they did or did not do caused their illness. One woman I know came out of surgery and said 'I'm sorry' to her husband. What was she sorry for? Getting breast cancer? You don't have to say you're sorry to anyone. You might have smoked a cigarette behind the school shed or drunk a glass of champagne or three on several occasions. Then again you might have exercised regularly all of your life, eaten only organic, been vegetarian, tea-total and kept your weight down. Either scenario still sees incidences of breast cancer. The point is, at this moment, we don't know what causes breast cancer. But we do know you can't blame yourself or anyone else. One belief that's commonly touted is that

> ## REMEDIES
>
> The Bach™ Flower essence pine is indicated for feelings of guilt. Like Rescue Remedy, pine works in a way that helps relieve the emotion of guilt so that you can view issues in a more positive light, thus helping you focus on healing.

certain personality types lead to breast cancer, however, a recent study shows that's baloney.

'Contrary to common belief personality traits such as neuroticism and extroversion do not determine a person's likelihood of developing cancer,' say Scandinavian researchers. The study was led by Dr Pernille Envold Hansen from the Danish Cancer Society in Copenhagen, Denmark, and found no indication of an association between personality traits and risks for cancer. However, the researchers concede it is still possible that personality traits coupled with a high-stress lifestyle may contribute.[99]

Fertility

If you are diagnosed with breast cancer and are still of reproductive age one of the issues you may be required to look at is the impact of treatment on your fertility. As breast cancer is more aggressive and is often found later when you are younger, treatment often includes chemotherapy or hormonal treatments which can send you into premature menopause. Or you may experience temporary menopausal symptoms like hot flushes, vaginal dryness and cessation of periods, which will revert to normal after 12 months. Your experience will depend on your individual treatment.

With regard to fertility women are born with a fixed number of eggs in our ovaries and breast cancer treatment could damage these irreparably. This raises a huge raft of issues, and if you were looking forward to having a family one day but have not yet done so, they are enormously difficult. If you already have children and had not planned on more, perhaps it won't be quite so hard to deal with.

If you have not yet had children and the idea of not being able to have them is devastating you could try speaking to Richard Fisher at Fertility Associates (see list of useful contacts on page 131). There has been enormous progress in the area of harvesting and storing eggs. There could be a possibility of removing your eggs prior to treatment and storing them until you are well. This does, however, raise all sorts of issues not least of which is the necessity of hormone treatment for egg retrieval. This could theoretically exacerbate the cancer. This is a highly specialised treatment and if you would like more information do give the experts a call. And after your breast cancer treatment is over? Would it be safe to have a baby if you are still fertile?

'It is safe if the woman is cured but we don't know for sure who is cured,' says Dr Link. 'Pregnancy does not cause recurrence but it could theoretically accelerate a relapse via the hormone stimulation of pregnancy if the woman is not cured. In saying that I've only seen this happen on two occasions in 25 years and I've seen dozens of women who have had children.'[100]

PREGNANCY-RELATED BREAST CANCER

These days more and more women are choosing to have children later in life. In fact, in New Zealand, the number of women having children between 35–45 years has doubled from ten per cent to 20 per cent since 1992. We have always seen breast cancers diagnosed during pregnancy and lactation, there is no data to suggest we are seeing more, but it does seem to make sense if we relate being older to an increased risk of getting the disease. Being diagnosed during this time, however, does raise some separate issues that warrant mention:

1. Breast cancer diagnosis can be delayed as breast symptoms are attributed to pregnancy or breast-feeding changes.

2. Being diagnosed at this time does not seem to impact on outcome.

3. Mammography is avoided during the first trimester, however, a lead apron can be used to shield the abdomen.

4. Ultrasound can be used safely throughout pregnancy.

5. Chemotherapy can be given safely after the first trimester.

6. Surgery can be undertaken during pregnancy, however, radiation therapy has to be delayed until after the baby is born.

Lymphoedema (swollen limb)

Lymphoedema is a swelling of the limb/s caused by a blockage of lymph flow through the lymphatic system. The lymph system or lymphatics as it's commonly called, is a poor cousin to the blood and circulatory system. Most people are unaware that it even exists, yet like all the organs and our systems it is no less important. This system is much like the circulatory system except it is lymph fluid that runs through the lymphatic vessels not blood.

Lymph is a clear fluid that drains waste products, toxins, pathogens and some cancer cells or, in simple terms, takes out the garbage. Lymphatic vessels lead to lymph nodes – tiny bean-shaped collections of immune cells of which there are about 600–1000 throughout the body. Lymph nodes contain specialised white blood cells called lymphocytes that can kill pathogens. The nodes can also trap cancer cells and slow them right down but, unfortunately, the nodes can sometimes be overpowered by them. Most of the lymphatic vessels that are found in the breast connect to the lymph nodes under the arms, known as axilla. (See the Breast diagram on page 18). If breast cancer (the villain) is on the move the first place you'll find it is here, which is why during breast cancer surgery the surgeon will examine whether or not cancer cells can be found in the axilla by removing several of the nodes or, in the case of sentinel node surgery (see Surgery on page 40) just the main draining one(s). For this reason a potential side effect of breast cancer surgery is a condition that can be a by-product of axilla removal called lymphoedema.

Lymphoedema is uncommon. If it does occur it will be minor or severe, i.e., the rings on your fingers might be tight or your arm may swell to three times its normal size. Lymphoedema may not show up for months or even years after surgery for breast cancer and if it does it is incurable. Caused by an accumulation of the lymphatic fluid it can cause your arm to feel uncomfortable, heavy, tight or stiff. Physical therapy using massage, compression, exercise and skincare can all help.

WHAT CAN YOU DO TO AVOID LYMPHOEDEMA?[101]

- Eat plenty of fruit and vegetables and drink lots of water to keep things flowing.
- Keep your weight down – this helps the lymphatic system.
- High temperatures can be aggravating because they induce further swelling so avoid hot baths, saunas, spas, hot pools and sunburn. However, some naturopaths will recommend certain treatments, including saunas, to induce sweating before or after lymphatic massage.
- Elevate the affected arm when you can.
- Apply lots of moisturiser because skin can become dry and flaky when the lymph is not flowing at optimum levels.
- Massage is good but is best left to someone who knows what they're doing. Heavy massage could be uncomfortable and damaging.
- Keep sleeves on garments loose and non-constrictive, and pad your bra strap.
- Avoid carrying heavy loads with the arm.
- Try to avoid injury as you may be more susceptible to infection.

Simplicité Fluid Cellulite Body Oil was originally created by herbalist David Lyons to get lymphatic drainage in the arm working after mastectomy and radiation.

- Be careful of insect bites.
- Use a file on fingernails rather than scissors.
- Wear gloves when doing chores and gardening.
- If you're sewing, wear a thimble – yes they do still exist!
- Treat cuts and scratches promptly by cleaning well and applying antiseptic.
- Use an electric razor for shaving under the arms.

Professional lymphatic massage is a massage technique that includes a gentle clearing of lymphatic node areas and a pumping motion of the body to clear fluid build up through the tissues. One of the best ways to promote circulation and support lymphatic flow is to stimulate the body through massage. You could see a naturopath to clear lymphatic blockages through massage clearing techniques. They will also show you how to maintain clear lymph flow through simple self-massage techniques that you can use 2–3 times daily. To give you a basic idea of how it is done, the lymph glands, stomach and chest area are massaged in a gentle pumping action, followed by the lymph node areas found under the arms, neck, behind the knees and the groin. After these areas have been gently pumped with the therapist's hands, the surface of the skin is massaged to encourage lymph flow and then the body is rocked side to side in a very small pumping–rocking motion. This treatment is a major priority to treat lymphoedema and must be practised by qualified health professionals aware of the contraindications with this massage.

Exercise can improve both blood and lymphatic circulation because the motion helps to move lymph fluid through the lymph vessels. Gentle trampoline bouncing improves lymphatic flow due to the movement similar to exercise and is especially recommended for those recovering from an illness. If you can't get the bounce going get someone else to gently bounce on the tramp at the same time.

Herbal extracts of sweet clover (*Mellilotus officinalis*), cleavers and self heal obtained from a naturopath or herbalist can be used to reduce congestion. This improves lymph flow by breaking down accumulated proteins.

Tissue cell salts are easily obtained from health stores and are very inexpensive. Nat Mur (sodium chloride) and Nat Sulph (sodium sulphate) are homeopathically prepared minerals that help to regulate and distribute body fluid more evenly. Take 1 tablet every 30 minutes for five days to help reduce symptoms rapidly, and then take at least 4 tablets of each mineral for 3–6 months. If you have a chat to the health store or pharmacy stockist you may find some of these tissue salts in one combined formula.

In your bath: A handful of Epsom salts (magnesium) or rock sea salt added to your bath for the last 15 minutes can aid removal of toxins and relax fatigued muscles.

Menopause

Menopause is something we all know we're going to go through at some stage. This is the time when periods stop and just when we think we're escaping from premenstrual syndrome and bloating we realise we're still going to experience mood swings, hot flushes and all sorts of other side effects. That's naturally occurring menopause. However, if it happens suddenly, as in the case of post-chemotherapy, it can seem like an added insult. Experiencing the diagnosis and treatment of breast cancer is hard enough to bear but if it means saying goodbye to the hope of having a baby as well as 'those' side effects, it can be devastating. You may experience weight gain, loss of libido, night sweats, problems sleeping and vaginal dryness as well. Once again, be kind to yourself and love yourself. There are ways to manage these symptoms and live more comfortably with menopause. Simple things to do when experiencing menopausal hot flushes include wearing layers (if you feel hot, you can peel the layers off to help you cool down) and wearing clothes made from natural fibres, such as cotton, as they tend to breathe a lot better than most synthetic materials. You could spray (spritz) cool water on your ankles and wrists (major pulse points) to help cool you down or apply a cool pack (damp face cloth) to your neck and forehead to provide relief. Sexual intercourse helps to increase circulation and keep the vagina lubricated and toned. But you may need a water-based lubricant to avoid irritating the vaginal walls. (See Sex on page 78 for more topical remedies.)

GOOD FOODS

At this stage what you need to do is to promote good oestrogen in your body, as good oestrogen can block bad oestrogen which may cause breast cancer to develop. Bad oestrogens include oestradiol, found in polyunsaturated and other fats, and chemical oestrogens, from pesticides.

Good oestrogens, such as plant oestrogens (also known as plant isoflavones and phyto-oestrogens [phyto means plant]) are found in soy foods as well as many herbs, plants and other food sources. Good oestrogens should also help lessen hot flushes and other menopausal symptoms. The following foods are all rich in plant oestrogens: soya textured vegetable protein (a mince substitute), tempeh, soy flour and flakes, soya vegetarian sausages, tofu, soy milk, flax seed (fresh seeds), buckwheat, millet, parsley, fennel, celery, sesame seeds, sunflower seeds, legumes, mung beans, sprouts and sprouted beans.

SUPPLEMENTS

Scientists have discovered why eating your greens is good for you. Certain herbs and vegetables contain powerful plant chemicals that have a protective effect against breast cancer and hormone sensitive tissues. To be more specific, if you eat cruciferous vegetables, such as broccoli, cabbage, Brussels sprouts and cauliflower, your risk of manifesting oestrogen sensitive cancers may be reduced. But to obtain this benefit you must eat large quantities of these raw vegetables daily.

As these greens are digested they are broken down into various by-products, including diindolylmethane (DIM) and indole-3-carbinol. DIM is a stable indole found in cruciferous vegetables, which promotes the healthy metabolism of oestrogen in both women and men. Because of its stability DIM is an excellent supplement: it changes the ratio of harmful oestrogen (16-hydroxy oestrogens) and beneficial oestrogen (2-hydroxy oestrogens) in the body, by producing more of the beneficial oestrogen. This is a sound strategy for reducing the risk for breast cancer.

Another potent herb that works to reduce the development of breast cancer is rosemary. Yes, besides working well with lamb roast, rosemary is a powerful antioxidant that can help inhibit breast cancer cells and can even enhance the effectiveness of certain cancer-fighting drugs to which some cancer cells can become resistant.

DIM (diindolylmethane) and **rosemary** (rosmarinic acid) can be safely taken during chemotherapy, while on Tamoxifen and for long-term general health maintenance. They are also recommended for those who suffer from hormonal migraines, have come off HRT, have a family history of breast cancer and those who have, or have had, breast cancer. Take 40mg of DIM twice daily and 50mg of rosemary twice daily.

Acidophilus and **bifidus** assist the body's conversion of phyto-oestrogens, which have beneficial effects on menopausal symptoms. Acidophilus and bifidus are available at most health food and nutrition stores and come in two forms – capsules and powder. Doses of acidophilus and bifidus preparations are based on the number of live bacteria. A common dose is 1–10 billion live bacteria, in divided doses, taken daily by mouth. Take 1 billion of acidophilus and bifidus species to repopulate your digestive system daily.

Wild yam, soy, red clover and **kudzu** are herbs that contain plant oestrogenic substances (isoflavones or phyto-oestrogens). As oestrogen levels decline women experience menopausal symptoms. By including more phyto-oestrogens in the diet these symptoms can be combated by fooling the body it has enough oestrogen.

Phyto-oestrogens can do this because they naturally mimic the body's oestrogen and are capable of binding to the cells' oestrogen receptors. To put it more simply, imagine a lock and a key. Each cell has a lock which can only be opened by a certain key. Once you open the lock the cell will behave in a different way.

Imagine the phyto-oestrogen as the key and the oestrogen receptor as the lock. Once the phyto-oestrogens have fitted into the oestrogen receptor the body's cells behave in ways that reduce menopausal hot flushes and vaginal dryness, help to protect bones, and even influence healthy cholesterol levels.

Other rich sources of plant oestrogens include flax seeds, nuts, whole grains, green soy beans (edamame), soy foods, apples, fennel, celery, parsley and sprouts, especially alfalfa. Including these in your diet is beneficial as well as supplementing with kudzu, red clover and soy extracts.

You may (or may not) want to have an Oestrogen Metabolism Assessment (see page 103 for full details) before taking phyto-oestrogen concentrated extracts or eating large amounts of phyto-oestrogenic foods. One more thing, give herbs time to work – it may take one to three months before you feel their beneficial effects.

To trick the body into thinking it has more oestrogen, therefore reducing menopausal symptoms, take 2g–4g of dried wild yam root three times daily, 2g–4g of red clover daily, 500mg of kudzu twice daily, 25mg of standardised isolated plant isoflavones soy extract daily. For best results use a combination of phyto-oestrogenic herbs, such as soy, red clover and kudzu mixed with black cohosh. This works far better for hot flushes and menopausal symptoms than using a single phyto-oestrogenic herb. Take up to the equivalent of 60mg of isolated phyto-oestrogens (plant isoflavones) daily from a combination of phyto-oestrogenic herbs or as professionally directed.

Other beneficial herbs which help combat menopausal symptoms include dong quai, sage, motherwort and black cohosh. These herbs, however, are not rich sources of phyto-oestrogens. They exert different actions on the body helping to reduce hot flushes, normalising heart palpitations and soothing the nerves and moodiness. Some women who cannot metabolise phyto-oestrogens into good oestrogens can use these herbs instead. (See Oestrogen Metabolism Assessment page 103.)

Dong quai used in combination with other herbs reduces the severity of hot flushes, insomnia, mood changes and vaginal dryness. Take 1g–2g daily.

Sage is famous for being an antihydrotic herb. This means it helps with night sweats, hot flushes and general excessive sweating brought on by heat or anxiety. Take 1g daily. If sage is taken over a long period of time it can cause vaginal dryness because of its astringent qualities. This is very rare and will only happen to a few women out of hundreds and can easily be counteracted with motherwort and yucca, which can be obtained through health stores, some pharmacies, naturopaths and herbalists.

Black cohosh is a herb that was historically used to treat mainly female conditions by native and early Americans. Since the 1950s German doctors have been recommending black cohosh for menopausal symptoms. Extensively researched, this valuable herb is used to treat sleep disturbances, headaches, hot flushes, increased perspiration, irritability and vaginal dryness. For years scientists and herbalists thought that black cohosh was a phyto-oestrogenic herb similar to soy or red clover, but recently this has been proved to be incorrect. Black cohosh reduces hot flushes relating to menopause by acting on temperature regulation through serotonin receptors in the brain rather than through its oestrogen-like effects as originally thought. For best results combine with the herbs motherwort and sage for day and night time sweats and insomnia. Take 1.5g–2g of black cohosh rhizome or root daily or 1mg of 27-deoxyactein (a standardised extract of the root and rhizome that proves to be very successful in clinical trials).

Motherwort soothes irritability, forgetfulness, moodiness and heart palpitations. This wonderful herb is great for us women who have need of a little mothering ourselves. Take 1g–2g daily.

Stress

You know the saying 'smile and the whole world smiles with you'. Without doubt it's a truism but sometimes life throws punches that make it damn hard to smile. Psychological stress and emotions have been known for some time to be associated with substantial physiological changes. Glucocorticoid chemicals are released in times of stress and can halt formation of new t-cells (part of the body's defence force), they can even cause them to commit suicide. Stress hormones are known to constrict the blood vessels and reduce the efficacy of the immune system. These adverse effects have raised questions as to whether stressful events can increase the risk of developing breast cancer.

While there have been many studies on the relationship of the two, the results have always been conflicting. A 15-year study conducted in Finland involving twins showed that severe stress (e.g., death of a spouse, separation/divorce, etc.) could increase the risk of developing breast cancer. However, what it didn't show is why. It could be that hormonal changes in the body caused by stress increase risk, or the way that stress impacts on diet, medication use and lifestyle habits, or it could be the way that stress affects the immune system.[102] Like so many causative theories relating to breast cancer, no one is certain about the relationship between stress and the disease.

Weight gain

Contrary to what many people think, weight gain can be a side effect of breast cancer treatment. Exercise is the key here, although if you're suffering from fatigue or depression that's the last thing you'll feel like doing. However, as you'll see in the following section, exercise won't only help you with weight gain, it can help with fatigue and depression also.

See a nutritionist or naturopath to help you with health and nutritional guidelines to lose weight. Steroid medication can cause weight gain so it is important to reduce weight through exercise and diet – only use health supplements with naturopathic and medical specialist supervision as some herbs, for example liquorice and ginseng, may increase the steroid medication's effects.

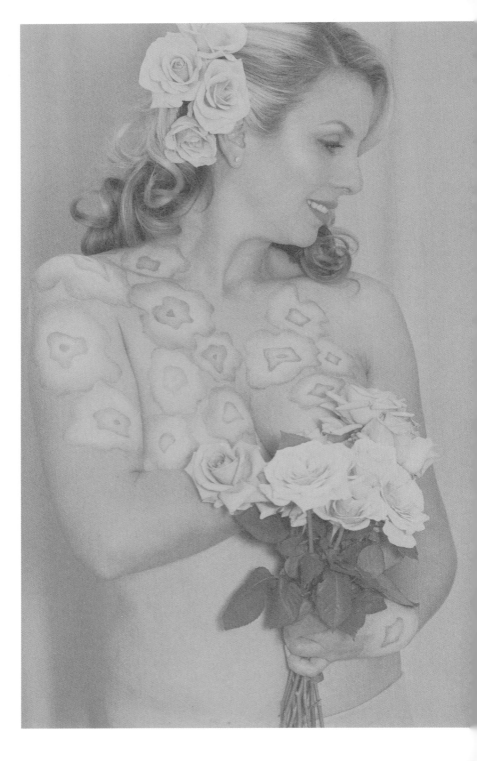

Relationships

Chances are your journey with breast cancer is going to affect your relationship with your partner, including your sex life. You're going to be looking at your body image, your femininity and your sexual attractiveness. And you will undoubtedly be harsh on yourself simply because you're a woman.

If you've had breast reconstruction you will still have visible breasts and if you've decided to go with prosthesis you will have the loss of one or both breasts to get used to. Either way you will have physical scars and you will look different from the woman you saw in the mirror before your experience with breast cancer.

Some people suggest standing in front of the mirror and picking out three things you like about yourself, first in your favourite outfit, second in lingerie and third stark naked. Then go through the same process with your partner. The thought behind the exercise is that it's important you both become familiar with your bodily changes.

These will be testing times for your relationship but the lovely thing is that what was a good relationship can become great – sharing tough times tends to do that. However, if your relationship wasn't so good it may lead to a few cracks. Mostly though you'll find your partner is there to support you and even though you may be thinking 'I'm damaged goods. What will he want with me?' He's probably thinking, 'I don't care about anything other than that you're here and I hate seeing you go through this trauma.' What's important to your partner is that the person they love is alive and doing well. Of course that doesn't mean there won't be ups and downs – this is the real world and ups and downs are part of everyday life. And if your relationship really was built on sand you may find one of you – and that could well be you – wants out.

Some women find that after having experienced a serious illness they want to make the most of their lives, which doesn't include an unfulfilling relationship. And sometimes a man just can't handle the stress. But statistically just as many women leave as men after an experience with breast cancer. How people react to a life challenge like this can differ greatly. In some it brings out their core strength, others find they don't cope very well at all and become fragile and vulnerable. But after riding it out, just like your hair, your spirit will usually come back. The ultimate would be to have a partner who is understanding and helpful and understands your change in demeanour. But some men just can't function through their own suffering. Some don't say anything much at all, not because they don't care but because they can't cope. But unhappily or happily, depending on how you look at it, breast cancer has become so common that most men have someone close in their life that has experienced the disease. There is absolutely no way to predict how any man will respond, but there is no doubt that many men are supportive and 'breaking up' is the furthest thing from their mind, whatever you might be thinking. As with any intimate relationship the secret to getting through is communication. Talking to each other, listening to each other and making time for each other is important. Often people feel lost. They don't know how to broach such a huge subject as cancer. Make a date with each other and talk about the little things until you can work up to the bigger picture. Try and get all your worries out into the open and let your partner do the same. This brings us rather neatly to sex.

Sex

Apart from your body-shape changes you'll probably notice other changes in yourself too, such as a decrease in libido, difficulty reaching orgasm and/or vaginal discomfort during sex. These are all big issues when it comes to your relationship. It's important you relax (which sounds like a very tall order considering everything you're dealing with). Bear in mind it is common to experience a decrease in sex drive after breast cancer treatment due to hormonal changes. Because breast cancer treatment works on reducing the female hormone levels – oestrogen, progesterone and testosterone – libido is affected. The female sex drive is actually driven by testosterone produced in the ovaries and adrenal glands (and we thought it was purely a guy-thing!). There are other side effects that could contribute to your not being in the mood too, such as fatigue and tenderness in the mouth and vagina. If not reaching orgasm is becoming an issue try not to focus on it (yes, difficult we know), instead concentrate on other things like kissing or massage. Fantasy is also a powerful tool – movies, erotica and sex toys, books and magazines.

It's not just the physical considerations you have to contend with, you've probably lost trust in your body and it feels vulnerable and fragile too. So is it any wonder you're experiencing some difficulty? If it's all just a bit too much, take the pressure off yourself and take it slow. If chemotherapy has led to vaginal dryness, try KY Jelly or Sylk lubricants (which you can pick up at the supermarket). Avoid Vaseline or hand cream as these are oil-based and can cause problems with infection. Your doctor can prescribe Ovestin (oestriol) in cream form or as a pessary, which contains a very small amount of oestrogen (not enough to be harmful) or Vagifem (oestradiol) a tablet which you place in your vagina which also contains a small amount of oestrogen. A non-hormonal option is Replens cream, however, it has limited availability in New Zealand. (The Cancer Information service might be able to let you know where you could get it. Call them on 0800 800 426.)[103] These creams and pessaries will help lubricate the vaginal tissues. If you're experiencing thrush, a common side effect of many medications, buy yourself some Canesten.

If you prefer to use natural alternatives some women use yoghurt (the plain variety or acidophilus) or olive oil. The yoghurt/olive oil devotees suggest using lots of it. (It might be wise to use a towel underneath and if you're using condoms don't go for the oil option – oil can alter the constitution of the condom.) Alternatively 10g of Manuka honey mixed with 100g of aqueous cream (obtained from a pharmacy) and 400IU of Vitamin E may help. Avoid antihistamines, alcohol and diuretics as these tend to dry up mucous membranes and the walls of the vagina. The herb yucca is also great for vaginal dryness.

Exercise has also been shown to have a positive effect on a person's sex life. Besides, toning and limbering up your muscles it will make you feel better about yourself. And speaking of exercise, you may want to try Kegel exercises. They may help with any decreased ability to orgasm that you are experiencing. To do them tense up as though you're stopping the flow of urine, then count to five, release and repeat. These can be done anywhere, anytime with no one being the wiser. They strengthen the pubococcygeal muscle in the lower vaginal area, which is the muscle that contracts during orgasm (also known as the love muscle).

The single girl

When Sally was first diagnosed with breast cancer her relationship with her then partner disintegrated. Not long after surgery and treatment she met Scott. She told him about her experience of breast cancer almost immediately and they are very happy today. The decision to tell or not to tell is always a struggle for a young single woman who has had breast cancer. She has all the 'normal' concerns like – will he think I'm pretty, will he think I'm nice, will he think I'm hot? However, in addition she has to wonder, 'Will he be turned off if he knows I'm scarred/missing a breast/have a reconstructed breast?' There's a myriad of issues to be dealt with. Another young woman met her partner just before she discovered she had breast cancer. They found the experience brought them closer and their love for each other was accelerated because of the illness. They were married just as soon as she felt her hair was long enough.

The important thing to remember is that you're still you. If you're sent into early menopause by your treatment it's difficult because it adds another hurdle to the obstacle course. You have to come to terms with your inability to have children. That by itself is something that can take a long time to accept. The dating game is never easy and singledom these days is common whether you've had breast cancer or not. The 'difficult dating' scenario is nothing to do with your illness but everything to do with the lives we lead today. It's harder to meet people. So go out with friends, be honest in your own time and know you are not defined by your illness. And put yourself in the guy's shoes. If he told you he had had testicular cancer, would you put him in the too-hard basket?

5 What you can do to reduce the risk of getting breast cancer

THERE ARE MANY WAYS you can find opportunities in your lifestyle to help prevent breast cancer. It would take a series of books to write down all the healthy things we could do but it's important to get a handle on a few basics. That said, none of us are saints and it's very difficult to be 100 per cent healthy 24/7. And, quite honestly, if we tried to rule out every one of the possible risks of breast cancer, life wouldn't be too much fun. One day, during the writing of this book, the pair of us sat at the table discussing this very subject. (Naturally it's on your mind when it's consuming your life!)

We were having lunch of a herbal tea and organic chickpea salad. It was very healthy and delicious too. However, we ended up very bloated from nasty chickpea gas so we saved ourselves by taking digestive enzymes. Let's face it, we were at a naturopath's home so all of these things were right on hand.

Later that night we dined at a Turkish restaurant and the conversation once again turned to what we were prepared to do or change in our diet to look after our breasts. This conversation took place over a yummy bottle of wine. We had to ask ourselves could we give up our wine, the occasional punnet of hot chips or bowl of ice-cream forever? Honestly, the answer was no. So we decided to adopt the 80:20 rule. We'd follow the rules 80 per cent of the time and do what we like the rest. Cheers to that!

Diet

We are what we eat. That truism has been around for many years and its accuracy could well explain its longevity. As much as 30 per cent of the breast cancer risk has been linked with the way we eat and there have been countless studies involving breast cancer and diet. Diet is important because it's one thing we really can control.

Women are continually asking Lani for advice on what to eat when they experience an illness. Often the doctor hasn't made any recommendations nutritionally. In actual fact doctors don't spend a lot of time at medical school studying nutrition so it's not generally a specialty of theirs. Good nutrition is often not taught properly in schools either so we tend to rely on TV programmes, books and friends to influence our eating choices.

Once again it's important to become informed. One of the tricks to healthy eating is finding out what the healthy foods are and learning how to cook and prepare these foods in healthy delicious ways.

THE FRUIT AND VEGETABLE DEBATE

Many organisations recommend seven to ten portions of fruit and vegetables a day for breast cancer patients (thoroughly washed please – we believe pesticides are a concern). However, a recent study of over quarter of a million women from ten different countries concluded that eating large amounts of fruit and vegetables has no effect on breast cancer risk.[104] Researchers were speechless because it contradicts a commonly held health belief. In the Harvard University Nurses' Health Study, researchers reported results that fruit and vegetable consumption is not significantly associated with reduced breast cancer risk.[105] Yet another study found that the consumption of vegetables, but not fruit, contributed to a reduction in breast cancer rates, and yet another found the risk of breast cancer declined with increasing the intake of dark yellow-orange vegetables, Chinese white turnips (the study was in Shanghai) and certain dark green vegetables.[106,107]

Hmmmm! Study results are confusing. But even if the results are correct in terms of breast cancer risk that doesn't mean eating a high proportion of fruit and vegetables should go low on your priority list. They make you feel good! And whatever the studies say, we're positive they contribute to wellbeing.

RAW POWER

Leslie Kenton, health guru and author of many books including *Raw Energy* and *The Powerhouse Diet*, believes you should eat loads of fruit and vegetables, preferably raw. Raw is another side to the debate – many fruit and vegetables lose a lot of their nutrients if they're cooked. 'Many physicians and healers have cured themselves of serious illness by eating a diet high in uncooked foods,' she says. She tells the story of a Danish physician, Kristine Nolfi, who turned to raw foods in a bid to beat her own breast cancer and won. 'Then she taught her patients about this natural form of healing. Her success was so great (as was the fury her treatments unleashed among her orthodox peers) that she gave up using drugs altogether and started the Humlegaarden Sanatorium in Denmark which she ran until her death in 1957.'

Leslie herself has long been a raw food eater after being healed of depression in her twenties by Dr Gordon Latto and Dr Phillip Kilsby – British GPs who believe that a raw regime stimulates the body to heal itself. 'The use of uncooked foods is growing. All over the world, "live" foods and juices are part of the gentle treatment of cancer,' says Leslie. 'Nevertheless the principles of healing underlying the use of raw foods are still foreign to the training doctors receive. Unfortunately, in most medical schools, no more than a couple of hours' training is given in nutrition. But the present health crises in the Western world and a growing demand for a "whole person" approach to health and illness continue to change all this. High-raw, low-grain eating is a way of living whose time has come.'[108]

'Live' fruit and vegetables contain a number of healthy, body-loving ingredients. **Carotenoids** are found in yellow and orange vegetables and fruits, and dark-green leafy vegetables. They include the sub-groups beta-carotene (high in kumara or sweet potato and carrots), lutein (abundant in spinach, parsley and kale) and lycopene (found in generous amounts in tomatoes).

Vitamin C or **Ascorbic acid** is a powerhouse of goodness and is abundant in citrus fruits and juices, tomatoes, melon, strawberries, broccoli and green leafy vegetables.

Vitamin E is another goody the body loves. Eat broccoli, olives, blueberries, avocado and nuts to get your fill.

Get your **folic acid** requirements from greens such as beans, asparagus, leafy vegetables and broccoli.

Dietary fibre is a must for overall good health. This includes both cereal and vegetable fibre. Most fruits and vegetables contain plenty of it especially broccoli (there's that superfood again!), apples, oranges and berries.

Dithiolthiones, glucosinolates, indole-3-carbinol and **sulforaphane** are anti-cancer food chemicals found within the cruciferous family and vegetables of the Brassica genus, such as cabbage, kale, broccoli, cauliflower, Brussels sprouts, radishes, turnips and watercress.

Phyto-oestrogens act like a weak version of the hormone oestrogen and that's a good thing. They do not raise levels of oestrogen in the body but, in fact, work to decrease it. Bean sprouts, soybeans and dried beans and peas provide phyto-oestrogens.

So, relating to breast cancer risk, how are these constituents found in fruits and vegetables beneficial?

Controlling cell division: Some carotenoids (not all) convert to Vitamin A in the body which can lead to good cell growth. As discussed in 'what is breast cancer' cancer cells just keep on dividing. Carotenoids interfere with this uncontrolled activity and have the ability to pull the cells into line.

Waging war on free radicals: Vitamins A, C and E are natural antioxidants which can neutralise free radicals. Free radicals are naturally present in the body but outside influences such as pollution and smoking can exacerbate them. They love to damage cells and generally wreak havoc in the body. The antioxidants can knock them dead.

Boosting the immune system: It's common knowledge that fruit and vegetables help fight against disease. It is now also thought that vitamin C is directly involved in the maintenance of the immune system by synthesising specific molecules, which aid in immunity function.

Normalising oestrogen levels: Phyto-oestrogens in plants can help decrease oestrogen levels in a woman's body and that's got to be a good thing as breast cancer is believed to be the result of oestrogen dominance in the body.

FIBRE

Modern Western diets contain much less fibre than is desirable. To raise the levels you need to start eating more fruit, vegetables, legumes and whole grains. This assists general health anyway, from bowel complaints to general bloating. Epidemiological studies have found that fibre intake from plants is protective against breast cancer (as well as other cancers), cardiovascular disease, diabetes and obesity – that's got to be a good thing.

FATS

Eat less animal fat.[109] Animal fat is a saturated fat (those that go hard at room temperature). Eating excessive amounts of animal fat is linked to an increase in breast cancer. One theory is that it's because pollutants and hormones that might trigger breast cancer are stored in animal fat. Another theory is that obesity is linked to breast cancer and people who are overweight tend to have high fat diets.

It's not as hard as you think to cut down on eating animal fat and cheese. There are wonderful low fat options and recipes available so your new low calorie diet is tasty and healthy. But reducing your overall saturated animal fat intake means eating less fried food, food cooked in lard, heated oils and fats, and solid fats (animal fats).

Substitute these with healthy oils. Olive, canola, soybean, safflower, peanut and avocado oils can be used in place of saturated animal fats. The bad news is that heating these oils and frying food destroys their beneficial qualities.

Flash fry your food instead of deep frying it to lessen the amount of heated fats you have in your diet. Heat the pan then add a teaspoon of oil (olive or avocado preferably). Then cook your meat or vegetables. Add a little water and use the steam to help cook your food. Other healthy methods of cooking include grilling, boiling or steaming. Another way to add these oils to your diet is to make homemade mayonnaise, aioli, and salad or vegetable oil dressings that you can add to your meal after it is cooked, giving it a creamy texture and flavour.

Essential fatty acids (EFA) are beneficial because the body requires omega 3 and 6 to function at an optimal level, and we cannot make these substances ourselves. We can obtain omega 3 and 6 essential oils from fish, hemp seed, soybean, walnut, safflower, sesame, flax seed oil, evening primrose oil, hemp oil and borage oil. You can add these to your diet without too much hassle as they are easy to come by in supplement form.

Flax seed, fish and evening primrose oil

The leading authority on dietary fats, Udo Erasmus, recommends a balanced ratio of dietary omega 3 and omega 6 fats. He says it's critical if you have breast cancer, or any form of cancer, and you're taking evening primrose oil (EPO) to take omega 3 rich fish or flax seed oil as well. EPO is rich in omega 6, but has no omega 3 essential fats. Although omega 6 is beneficial for PMS, lumpy breasts and menopausal symptoms, according to Erasmus, too much omega 6 enhances tumour formation and growth, while omega 3 inhibits tumours.[110] Many people are deficient in omega 3, more so than omega 6 because we tend to have more omega 6 vegetable oils in our diet. You don't need to stop taking omega 6 altogether, just combine it properly with omega 3 oils. Fresh fish oil and flax seed oil are excellent rich sources of omega 3. Other sources include seafood, salmon, eel, mackerel, trout, tuna, sardines and snapper. If you like fish, eat fresh fish at least three times a week. It's best not to fry the fish but to eat it raw, sashimi style, or to steam or boil it, whole or filleted, with the skin on. As Erasmus reminds us 'the oils we want are found under the skin, especially behind the gills, around the fins and along the belly'.[111] Other options include the tinned fish varieties. If you don't like fish, supplement with 3000mg of omega 3 capsules daily or 1 tablespoon of flax seed oil daily.

Our personal favourite is flax seed oil because it contains omega 3, 6 and 9. And it's simple to include in your diet by taking 1–2 tablespoons per day. Flax seed oil connoisseurs can take it directly from a tablespoon or if you enjoy munching on scrumptious salads, substitute the olive oil for flax seed oil and mix it with lime, garlic, lemon juice or balsamic vinegar for a delicious salad dressing. Besides these tasty dressings, flax seed oil can be mixed into smoothies, mayonnaise, butter, yoghurt or drizzled over vegetables, toast and baked potatoes. It's important not to heat or fry flax seed oil, as it will spoil due to its fragility. And if you keep it refrigerated once opened, you can use it for up to three months.

ALCOHOL

For many of us drinking a beer or glass of wine after a busy day is soothing to the nerves. But more than two standard glasses per day may lead to an increase of circulating oestrogen levels and an increased risk of breast cancer. Alcohol may also dramatically increase the amount of 'bad oestrogen' in your body if you're taking HRT. If you like alcohol, stick to two or less standard servings a day. A standard serve of wine with an alcohol content of 12–14 per cent is roughly 100ml. Other examples of standard servings of beverages include one 300ml glass of beer or one 25ml measure of spirits. Red wine has a reputation for being high in antioxidants and protective for the heart and blood vessels – good news for all you red wine lovers. But if you're thinking of not drinking Monday to Friday then polishing off a bottle of wine and a couple of beers on a

Saturday, think again. Just because you have missed out on a potential ten servings of alcohol by Friday doesn't mean you can lump them all together at dinner on Saturday or Sunday. Good try though! Like us, you're probably not perfect and will overindulge every now and then, we've all gotta live. Remember the 80:20 rule.

FOODS AND NUTRIENTS THAT PROTECT YOU FROM BAD OESTROGEN

Breast cancer is linked to an overproduction of oestrogen of which there are two types – the good oestrogen and the bad oestrogen (see page 29). Your diet can help fight the bad guy.

Cruciferous vegetables: Indole-3-carbinol and sulforaphane are found in the cruciferous family of vegetables: broccoli, cauliflower, cabbage, Brussels sprouts and kale. Scientific studies show that adding these vegetables to your diet can help prevent certain forms of cancer including breast cancer.[112] Another good reason to eat your Brussels sprouts! If you're not keen on too many fibrous greens you can buy powdered green foods from your health store. They're normally a combination of Spirulina, chlorella, broccoli and vitamin C. Just add a teaspoon to a smoothie or have a 'shot' drink of greens in the morning mixed with cold water.

Indole-3-carbinol helps the breakdown of oestrogen into 'good' guys rather than 'bad' guys. Diindolylmethane (DIM) is one of the few supplements available over the counter that, as a natural indole supplement, improves the way the body breaks down oestrogen. It also helps the body turn oestrogen into a healthy oestrogen metabolite (2-hydroxyestrone). Take 40mg–200mg daily. DIM is also helpful for hormonal-induced headaches and migraines and some women find it helpful for menopausal hot flushes taken alongside phyto-oestrogenic herbs.

Fresh flax seed, aka linseed, is easily found at health stores. A coffee grinder (or mortar and pestle) are the ideal way to grind these seeds up to sprinkle onto your breakfast or add to yoghurt, shakes or salad dressings. Alternatively you could smash them up in a plastic bag using a rolling pin. Another good way to eat them is to mix linseed (L), sunflower seeds (S) and almonds (A). These make up the popular LSA mix many people are using as a food sprinkle. Flax seeds are rich in omega 3 and almond and sunflower seeds are rich in omega 6, so LSA gives you a well-balanced mix. Other omega 6 rich nuts include brazil nuts and walnuts. Flax seeds have a delicious, fresh nutty taste and supply beneficial lignans. The lignans compete with bad oestrogen on breast cell sites, giving a protective effect. Flax seed has a natural laxative action as well because it supplies a lot of fibre in addition to small amounts of omega 3, 6 and 9. One to three teaspoons per day is adequate.

> LSA can be stored in the freezer.

Lignans are compounds found in some (though not all) plants. Research facilities, including the University of Toronto, Canada, have discovered that plant lignans have immunomodulating or immune-balancing properties. Flax seed fibre is one of the richest sources of lignans. Whole grains and rye also supply lignans. A decrease in protective lignans is linked to the low fibre intake in many Western diets and a rise in colon, breast and prostate conditions. They have been shown to have protective phyto-oestrogenic properties, helping the balance of hormones within the body and also possess natural antioxidant actions. Lignans have also been shown to exert anti-viral, anti-fungal and anti-cancer activities.

Phyto-oestrogens are believed to bind with oestrogen receptors in the body, competing with the body's natural oestrogens and other hormones for these sites found on the breast, cervix, colon and prostate. In simple terms they help to prevent the growth of hormone-based tumours and growths, while helping the body get rid of excess bad oestrogen. Phyto-oestrogens have therefore been associated with a decrease in hormone dependant tumours (as in some types of breast cancers). Phyto-oestrogens can also provide good oestrogenic stimuli in the absence of sufficient natural oestrogen in the body and are of benefit in assisting with some menopausal symptoms, e.g., hot flushes. Phyto-oestrogenic rich herbs and foods include red clover and kudzu and nuts, seeds and legumes, e.g., alfalfa sprouts, sprouted legumes and fermented soy products.

Rosemary has wonderful natural antioxidant, protective properties against oestrogenic tumours and may improve poor circulation and digestion. It may also enhance your body's metabolism of 2-hydroxy oestrogens ('good' oestrogens) and reduce 'bad' oestrogens (4-hydroxy oestrogen and 16-hydroxy oestrogen).

Seaweed: Nori, Japanese seaweed and kelp could also provide protection against breast cancer. Many health books hypothesise that traditional Japanese diets are linked with the low breast cancer rates in Japan. The Japanese have long appreciated the use of iodine-rich seaweed as an everyday food. Seaweed contains a rich store of minerals, particularly iodine, which is used by the thyroid gland. Iodine is used to make the hormone thyroxine, which is responsible for basal metabolic rate and carbohydrate/lipid/protein metabolism and other functions of the body.

Iodine: A Canadian pharmacology professor and general practitioner, Dr David Derry, who has been practising as a family doctor in Victoria, Canada, for the last 25 years, has been prescribing female patients 5ml–10ml of Lugol's iodine in juice per day.

In 1993 the *Canadian Journal of Surgery* described the benefits of iodine in reducing and removing fibrocystic breast lumps. Dr Derry became intrigued by this report and although the iodine therapy may take anywhere from two months to two years for the complete disappearance of breast lumps, the success rate so far has been 100 per cent. Derry is adamant that most women do not get nearly enough iodine in their diet to protect their breasts against lump formation and also believes that a lack of iodine may be an important risk factor for breast cancer.[113]

New Zealand has a very low level of iodine in the soil in many areas, and recently there has been a rise in iodine deficiencies.[114] Low iodine levels also contribute to obesity. The blame is pointing to the increased use of non-iodised gourmet salt (celtic, rock and unprocessed sea salt), as people are cutting back on iodised table salt. Doctors are reluctant to recommend iodine (Lugol's) and kelp tablets because, while adverse effects of a high intake are unlikely when the thyroid gland is healthy, those who habitually have a low intake as well as those with abnormalities of the thyroid gland may respond adversely.[115] We recommend including Japanese seaweed cuisine in your diet. If seaweed isn't to your taste, use Lugol's to boost your levels of iodine. Talk to your health professional before taking these supplements and ask your health professional to monitor and supervise you if you take Lugol's or kelp tablets or if you suspect a thyroid condition.

Antioxidants are found in a large variety of fruits, vegetables, nuts, seeds, some minerals and protein. The best news of all is that they have natural anti-cancer properties. Damage from free radicals and toxins can lead to the cells' DNA (the cells' blueprint or map) receiving mixed messages. Once a mixed message is received the cell can lose control over its rate of growth and function, leading to cancer. Antioxidants prevent and reduce free radical-induced damage and offer protection against the growth of breast cancer cells. These wonderful antioxidants can be found in fruits, seeds, meat and vegetables. Incorporate a wide variety of these in your diet.

Vitamin C rich foods include kiwifruits, citrus fruits such as oranges, lemons, tangerines, grapefruit, etc., cranberries, blackcurrants, strawberries, cherries, tomatoes, papaya, capsicums and green leafy vegetables.

Cruciferous vegetables such as cabbage, broccoli, Brussels sprouts and cauliflower have antioxidant capabilities because of their high vitamin C content and flavonoid content. They also contain plant chemicals called indoles and isocyanates that help cells detoxify chemical carcinogens.

The onion family: garlic, onions, shallots, spring onions and leeks contain flavonoids, vitamin C, selenium and sulphur-containing substances. Observations in Italy and China show an association between a high consumption of garlic and onions and low rates of cancer.

Carotenoids These potent phyto-chemicals (plant chemicals) are the fat-soluble pigments abundant in yellow, orange, red and green fruits and vegetables. Beta-carotene and related carotene foods include **Spirulina**, carrots, squash, yams, sweet potatoes and apricots. Alpha carotene and lutein are present in green leafy vegetables and lycopene in tomatoes.

Selenium foods include garlic, onions, shallots, leeks, asparagus, seafood and fish, meats, brewers yeast, wheat germ and bran, whole grains and sesame seeds.

Zinc is found in rich supply in pumpkin, sunflower seeds, meats, oysters and other seafood.

Manganese is present in whole grains, green leafy vegetables, legumes, nuts, pineapples and egg yolks.

Methionine and **cysteine** sources include beans, fish, liver, eggs, brewers yeast and nuts.

Flavonoid rich foods include grapes, blueberries (also known as bilberry, it provides antioxidant anthocyanidins), strawberries, other berries (especially those that are blue or red), plums, capsicums and other foods with red, blue, violet or yellow plant pigments.

CALORIC RESTRICTION MAY LESSEN THE RISK OF BREAST CANCER[116]

We know that maintaining a healthy weight reduces our risk of cancer while obesity increases the risk, especially if we tend to hold weight around our middle. But what type of calorie restriction are we talking about? We've talked about eating less animal fat, but what about sugar? If we eat too much sugar this also raises our overall calorie consumption. However, apart from calories, sugar may pose a graver risk.

Does sugar feed cancer?
There is a saying often bandied around in nutrition circles that 'sugar feeds cancer'. Back in the 1930s Otto Warburg discovered that malignant tumours require glucose (sugar) to grow.[117] That's not so surprising as all of our cells need a certain amount of glucose. What was of significance was that the cancer cells required four to five times more glucose than normal cells. Without glucose cancer cells can't divide so rapidly. So significant was this discovery that Warburg was awarded the 1931 Nobel Laureate.

Patrick Quillin, the director of nutrition for Cancer Treatment Centers of America in Tulsa, Oklahoma, says he is puzzled as to why this is so overlooked as part of a comprehensive cancer treatment plan. 'Most patients I work with have a complete lack of nutritional advice,' he says. 'I believe many cancer patients would have a major improvement in their outcome if they controlled the supply of cancer's preferred fuel, glucose. By slowing the cancer's growth, patients allow their immune systems and medical therapies such as chemotherapy, radiation and surgery to reduce the bulk of the tumour mass to catch up to the disease. Controlling one's blood-glucose levels through diet, supplements, exercise, meditation and prescription drugs when necessary can be one of the most crucial components to a cancer recovery program.'[118,119,120]

It's been 74 years and not everyone is in agreement. One case study carried out in Italy of 2567 women with breast cancer discovered that they ate more high glycaemic index (GI) foods (e.g., white bread) than the control group of 2588 women who had no breast cancer. The control group ate a diet of predominanatly medium GI foods (e.g., pasta). This suggests a possible link between eating high GI foods and an increase in the development of breast cancer risk. Consequently, researchers go on to suggest that insulin resistance may play a role in the development of breast cancer.[121] A five-year U.S. study of over 60,000 women found no association between dietary glycaemic load and breast cancer risk making the relevance of such dietary patterns for breast cancer risk unclear.[122] At present, what we can be sure of is that maintaining a healthy weight by healthy means lowers the risk for breast, colon, pancreatic, ovarian and endometrial cancer, and other health related-issues.[123,124,125,126]

So if you can identify with what Patrick Quillin is saying you could adopt a long-term eating plan that helps to control blood glucose. It's actually quite easy cooking creative tasty meals from foods that have a low glycaemic load. Even Lani's fifteen-year-old step-daughter who only a year ago couldn't put a salad together taught herself to cook great, healthy balanced meals in a matter of weeks. John Ratcliff authored a book called *Low Carb Made Easy*.[127] We think it puts together the idea of a low glycaemic diet with recipes in an easy to read manner.

TO SOY OR NOT TO SOY

Soy has gained a controversial reputation over the years. But it has also had an upsurge in popularity. Soy lattes and flat whites taste great, but are they OK on a regular basis, if at all?

Soy beans are used in a variety of foods and supplements because they yield protein, fibre, a little fat and phyto-oestrogens. They're found in various forms in foods including milk, bread and even sausages. Natural HRT replacements combine soy with other herbs to stop menopausal hot flushing because when oestrogen levels are low soy can mimic oestrogen. It's many times weaker than the oestrogen the body makes and therefore deemed safer.

Advertisers expound the benefits of soy milk compared to cows' milk as it has no cholesterol, is low in fat and offers a tasty alternative. It even comes in a range of flavours: vanilla, strawberry, banana, cappuccino and chocolate. So, what's not to love about soy?

Strong evidence suggests that consumption of soy is breast cancer protective. Studies show that it can stop growth of breast cancer cells and it can lower the levels of harmful oestrogens within the body.[128,129] To support this theory some human and laboratory studies have proposed that in Asian countries, where the consumption of soy and plant-based oestrogens is considerably higher than in Western countries, the risk of breast cancer is reduced. This is because the incidence of breast cancer is lower in Asian countries than in Western countries.

Also, if Asian women and men migrate and adopt typical Western lifestyles and diet, their rate of breast and prostate cancer increases.[130] However, you could also argue that Asian diets tend to be high in fibre, vegetables and low in meat and animal fat compared to Western diets. This reduces possible risk factors for developing certain types of cancer.

So what's the controversy? While some studies have found that high doses of the antioxidant isoflavone genistein found in soy have stopped the growth of breast cancer cells, in other studies (*in vitro* and *in vivo*) low doses have been shown to stimulate cancer cells.[131,132] (*In vitro* refers to an experiment 'in glass', i.e., in a test tube or in the laboratory; *in vivo* means the test is done on a living organism.)

Where does that leave us as consumers? Perhaps a cautious approach should be taken when adding soy to the diet. See a naturopath if you:
- want to consume soy and are worried about its impact on your health;
- have breast cancer;
- have had breast cancer;
- have a genetic link to breast cancer;
- have menopause and want to use phyto-oestrogens and soy HRT replacements;[133] or
- have a vegetarian diet and rely on soy as a daily protein replacement.[134]

See a naturopath also for a diagnostic test called the Oestrogen Metabolism Assessment, which will discover how you metabolise oestrogen. It can give you an idea of whether you metabolise oestrogens into 'good' or 'bad' oestrogen metabolites. Once given the all clear, consume soy to your heart's content in balanced meals and focus on all the health benefits you could be getting from soy. The assessment is performed by Great Smokies Diagnostic Laboratory (GSDL) in America. The naturopath sends a sample of your urine to the GSDL for testing.

If you want to learn more about soy, phyto-oestrogens and recipes, authors Sue Radd and Dr Kenneth Setchell have written *Eat to Live*, it's a great book and you don't need a degree to understand it.

Soy consumption, beyond the breast
Uncooked soy protein has a goitrogenic effect which means that it may have a negative impact on a healthy thyroid gland and lower its function and your metabolism. So make sure your soy beans, tempeh, tofu, textured vegetable protein or whatever shape or form your soy comes in is cooked or fermented. If you have a hyper thyroid condition have your thyroid hormone levels regularly checked if you eat soy or take soy supplements. Avoid it altogether if your thyroid function lowers. You can talk to your naturopath and endocrinologist for more information, treatment, support and monitoring of the thyroid gland if needed.

Soy sources
You can add soy to your diet by incorporating different products in your meals. The following are all available in soy varieties: bread, cereal, cheese, edamame (green soy bean), flour, hot dogs, milk, miso, soy nuts, protein bars, protein powders, sausages, soybean sprouts, tamari, tempeh, textured vegetable protein, tofu (firm and soft) and yoghurt.

SUPPLEMENTS

Now that you're aware of what to avoid and what to add to your diet, it's time to boost your nutrition with supplements. Some of the possible supplements we've mentioned are kelp, iodine, soy, omega 3 (fish oil or flax seed oil), fibre (flax seed fibre, vegetables), DIM, evening primrose oil, green tea, antioxidants, vitamins and minerals.

What a mouthful! 'Should I take all of them at once,' you may be asking in horror! No, don't worry. What's probably more important is consistency with a few supplements rather than arming yourself with hundreds of supplements and only taking them diligently for about a month. You could have a personal consultation with a naturopath who can create a supplement programme specifically for you. Or you could choose your own with your new empowered knowledge. We don't want to load you up with too many supplements so here are a few basics that can help protect your body and upgrade your nutritional defences.

Coenzyme Q10 (ubiquinone): A potent antioxidant and natural compound found in the body. It also plays an important role in cellular energy production, immune function and cardiac protection. A deficiency of CoQ10 can affect DNA synthesis and promote cell mutations. Take 75mg daily.

Multivitamin and mineral supplements: You need an optimal intake of nutrients if you want your body to repair, heal and regenerate itself properly. Multis supply a great deal of the nutrients in one tablet. That's why they're pretty chunky most of the time, unless you find a suitable liquid variety. Keep in mind that some nutrients found in a multi will be ample, others won't be. It depends on your individual needs. New Zealanders have been found to be particularly deficient in vitamins C, E, B1, B2, B12, folic acid, calcium, iron, zinc and selenium. These nutrients are important for immune function, prevention of cancer, healthy tissues (nerve, bones and the heart), proper blood and cell formation and brain and kidney function.

Permitted forms and RDI of vitamins and minerals
It's important to choose a multi that is stronger than the recommended daily intake (RDI), as these are really a recommendation of a dose that you would need at minimum levels. By taking a high potency multi you can ensure that you are helping to correct micronutrient deficiencies for nutritional health insurance. Although try not to be lulled into a false sense of security and justify irresponsible eating, because the vitamin supplement will not meet all your nutritional needs. Healthy eating, drinking and lifestyle are important too.

5 | REDUCING THE RISK

We've included a table to give you some guidelines as to the RDI of vitamins and minerals.

VITAMIN OR MINERAL	RECOMMENDED DAILY INTAKE
Vitamin A	4000IU–5000IU or 750mcg retinal equivalents
Vitamin D	400IU or 10mcg cholecalciferol equivalents
Vitamin E	15IU or 10mg a-tocopheryl equivalents 50IU (if menopausal)
Vitamin K	Multis don't normally include this nutrient*
Vitamin B1 (thiamine)	1.1mg
Vitamin B2 (riboflavin)	1.7mg
Vitamin B3 (niacin or nicotinamide)	10mg
Vitamin B5 (pantothenic acid)	A minimum requirement of 10mg–15mg has been suggested*
Vitamin B6 (pyridoxine)	2mg
Vitamin B12 (cyanocobalamin)	2mcg
Folic acid (folate)	200mcg–300mcg
Other B complex vitamins include biotin, choline, inositol and PABA – B13 (orotic acid) B15 (pangamic acid) and B17 (amygdalin/laetrile).	Choline, biotin and inositol can be found in multis in a variety of doses*
Vitamin C	40mg
Magnesium	320mg
Calcium	800mg
Chloride	Multis don't normally include this nutrient*
Sulphur	Multis don't normally include this nutrient*
Sodium (salt)	Multis don't normally include this nutrient*
Phosphorus	1000mg – Multis don't normally include this nutrient
Potassium	Multis don't normally include this nutrient*
Chromium	A minimum requirement of 150mcg has been suggested*
Copper	Look for a multi that contains 1mg of copper per 10mg of zinc*
Fluoride	Multis don't normally include this nutrient*
Iodine	150mcg (maximum amount allowable 300mcg)
Iron	12mg
Manganese	A minimum requirement of 10mg has been suggested*
Selenium	A minimum requirement of 30mcg has been suggested*
Zinc	12mg

* *No RDI has been established. Sourced from NZ Consolidated Food Regulations 1998.*

Now that you are aware of the RDIs, look for a multi that contains a more potent amount of vitamins and minerals especially vitamin C, E, B1, B2, B12, folic acid, calcium, iron, zinc and selenium. Talk to your health professional or health expert if you don't know which multi to choose. Health stores and pharmacies have excellent trained staff and access to free naturopathic advice lines from supplement manufacturers.

Desirable supplements
- **Multi vitamin and mineral formula** Take one a day.
- **Antioxidant formulas** Choose a full spectrum formula. One that includes green tea, polyphenols, grape seed, pine bark, beta-carotene, vitamins E, A and C, proanthocyanidins, flavonoids and adjunctive minerals (zinc, selenium, manganese and iron). You can find antioxidant supplements that already contain one or more of these antioxidants.
- **Coenzyme Q10** Take 75mg daily.
- **Fish or flax seed oil** Take 3000mg daily.
- **DIM** (Diindolylmethane) Take 40mg–200mg daily.
- **Herbal detoxes** We know that environmental toxins are on the rise, so you must protect your body and help it cleanse and regenerate. Ask at your health store or pharmacy or see a naturopath to provide a detox herbal formula that at least includes milk thistle, chlorella, burdock root and red clover. You may like to do a seven-day, 14-day or one-month detox. You should complete these once or twice a year.

THE BEST DIET

This list will help you to summarise key health food choices to incorporate in your daily diet. Avoid any of these foods if you have sensitivities. If you want a personalised diet to suit you see a naturopath or nutritionist to give you alternatives and further guidelines.

- **Kelp** Combine ½ teaspoon with oil and lemon as a dressing, and add to vegetables, meat or salad.
- **Seeds and nuts** Linseeds (flax seeds), sunflower seeds, almonds or walnuts. Freshly crush and add 1–2 teaspoons to cereal, salad dressing or in protein shakes.
- **Oils** Avocado, olive, flax seed and evening primrose oil. You can heat avocado oil and olive oil but not the latter two. Take 1 teaspoon to 3 tablespoons of flax seed oil daily. Cook with 1–4 teaspoons of olive oil or avocado oil daily.

- **Fruit and vegetables** Eat a variety of vegetables, at least 3 cups daily and 2–4 pieces of fruit daily. Try making fruit and vegetable salsas to make meat meals tasty. You can also add more vegetables to stews, soups and puréed sauces.
- **Lean meat, fish and seafood** Eat 200g–600g daily depending on your needs and other types of protein you add to your daily diet.
- **Beans, legumes and soy products** Eat 200g–600g daily depending on your needs and other types of protein you add to your daily diet. Add a can of chickpeas or legumes to a chicken meal (curry) or add sprouts to your salad and soups.
- **Dairy** You can replace dairy with calcium-fortified soy milk, cheese and yoghurt. Or include small amounts of dairy products in your daily diet.
- **Whole-grain cereals** Eat whole grain cereals or rye rather than refined grains such as white flour products. Eat 200g–600g daily depending on your needs and the other types of carbohydrate you add to your daily diet.

CONCLUSION

The plain, down-to-earth, non-scientific or backed-by-studies truth is if you eat more uncooked fruit and vegetables, lower your grain and dairy intake and don't forget to include protein, you feel better, gain more energy, lose your desire for so-called 'undesirable' foods and you will feel more inclined to exercise. That's got to be good for you.

What we're advised to reduce, or avoid, are sugar, refined carbohydrates, caffeine, alcohol, red meats and dairy products as all of these foods have been associated with an increased risk of cancer.

Exercise

Exercise has been proven to be beneficial in both the prevention and treatment of breast cancer. Experts are also saying it can have a positive influence on breast cancer incidence as early-on as physical education classes at school (so get your daughters moving). It also helps with osteoporosis and heart disease, so starting early and creating a lifelong exercise habit can only be a good thing. In a 2003 study, women who exercised regularly from as young as 16 almost halved their risk of developing breast cancer after menopause, compared to women who had done no exercise.[135] 'Encore', an exercise programme run by the YWCA that gets phenomenally good results in America and Australia, is starting in New Zealand very soon. The programme runs once a week over eight weeks and is specifically for people who have had breast cancer surgery at any time in their lives. It involves two hours of pool and floor exercises followed by an inspirational speaker. Shelley Hannah, who instigated the New Zealand programme along with the YWCA's Di Paton, swears her competitive swimming (not to mention her passion for the sport) saved her from the pain and fatigue many women experience after breast cancer surgery. If she got into the pool and swam everyday she'd be pain-free but if for some reason she couldn't, the pain would reappear. Consistent correct exercise maintains healthy weight, reduces obesity and most importantly reduces the risk of developing breast cancer.[136,137] Different types of exercise methods are available from gentle harmonic yoga and more vigorous types of yoga and Pilates to swimming, weights, jogging, power-walking and dancing. Whatever your fancy, maintaining a healthy weight for your age and height and even restricting calories if necessary will lower your risk of breast cancer and other health conditions improving overall wellbeing. In actual fact, exercise is just as important as having a mammogram or checking for abnormalities.

> It has been suggested that exercising for 40 minutes, three times per week may reduce the risk of breast cancer by 20 per cent.

Things to avoid in the fight against breast cancer

There are certain things it might pay you to be cautious of in the world today when it comes to your health. Many of these things are controversial and not all are proven but they do add some food for thought and are something to be aware of.

SMOKING

Most people start smoking when they're young because they think it looks grown up and impressive. Pretty soon addiction or habits are set up and people find it hard to quit even though they know deep down it's not healthy or cool. If you think the health warnings on packets are for other people, it's time to stop kidding yourself.

Smoking causes cancer. Can you believe that studies on smoking, exposure to second-hand smoke and their link to breast cancer are controversial and inconclusive? Scientists are still not entirely sure that smoking leads to breast cancer. Good news for those who have hidden behind the bike shed for a fag. As a naturopath, the best advice I can give you is not to smoke. Perhaps deep down inside you agree too. If you smoke, want to be healthy, and if your focus is on preventing breast cancer, you will need to quit. Don't even think about smoking socially or sneaking out for the odd one, it doesn't work that way. The poisons in cigarettes leach into your cells robbing them of nutrients, energy and oxygen. It's not easy but they say it takes three weeks to make a habit and three weeks to break a habit. Treat your body with love and your body will look after you.

Still not convinced? If you still have the urge to smoke and aren't prepared to give up just yet, eat a balanced, high-fibre, healthy diet, rich in fruits, vegetables and whole grains. Take antioxidants, B vitamins and vitamin C daily. A lot of our friends who smoke have extremely healthy diets to help counteract the damage of smoking. Although not ideal, that's a great start. Smoking reduces the levels of a number of vitamins in your body. Taken daily, folic acid (400mcg), B complex vitamins, and the antioxidants vitamins E (400IU) and C (500mg–1000mg), and selenium (55mcg–100mcg) may improve lung function and protect you from lung cancer. Beta carotene, another well-known antioxidant and precursor to vitamin A, has been associated in more than one study with higher rates of lung and colon cancer in smokers who also drink alcohol. This may suggest that you avoid any formulas with beta carotene and rely on getting vitamin A from your foods until the studies are more conclusive in the safety and use of beta carotene for smokers who drink alcohol.

Use herbs to help your liver's detoxification processes to prevent liver and cellular damage. Milk thistle and dandelion root are marvellous liver-protecting herbs. You could also consider undergoing a gentle herbal detox twice a year.

RADIATION

Ionising radiation: Chest x-rays are performed to determine the health of the bones in the chest, the lungs, the heart and surrounding blood and lymph vessels. Radiation therapy has also been used to shrink the thymus, treat chest acne and of course treat certain type of cancers. Exposure to chest x-rays or radiation can damage the DNA of our breast cells. It's important to consider other forms of diagnosis or treatment before submitting yourself to a chest x-ray. However, if radiation diagnosis or treatment is a must, take antioxidants and include seaweed or iodine in your diet for the next three to five years to protect your DNA and ultimately your cells after a run of radiation treatment, or take them for at least six months after an x-ray diagnosis. Talk to a health care professional about the pros and cons of x-ray treatment to your breast area.[138]

UV radiation: The implications of other types of radiation are poorly understood, but we do know that excessive exposure to ultra violet rays including sun radiation, tanning and sun-beds should be avoided. Wear appropriate sun block and sunglasses when spending extended periods of time under the sun; this may help to reduce cataracts, skin damage, wrinkles and skin cancers. If you are determined to expose yourself to the strong rays of the New Zealand sun, make sure you don't get burnt. The more times you get sunburnt the higher your risk of melanoma will be.

Other radiation sources include microwave radiation, exposure during long airplane flights (over eight hours), TV, VDU computer screens, x-rays, radiation-therapy and mobile phones. Electromagnetic fields and radio frequency radiation is being investigated as a possible contributor to the development of breast cancer. We don't know for sure if living near great big, ugly power lines or transmitters will cause disease, but it's something to think about. Carotene and antioxidant supplements help prevent radiation damage. One of the top three supplements Lani always recommends is an antioxidant formula. Although you may not be able to instantly see or feel benefits from taking antioxidants, they are an important part of overall cell protection.

ENVIRONMENTAL FACTORS

The environment is everything around you. The air you breathe and the unseen chemicals in it, the water you drink, the chemicals you put on your skin and inhale from cosmetics, hair dyes, household cleaning products, cars, industrial pollution (and the list goes on) can all have an impact on your health.[139] Those who live in the city have a higher exposure to industrial and car exhaust pollution than those who live rurally. Organic produce is a healthier option because it's not loaded with pesticides or had chemicals added to prolong the shelf life and they generally taste better.

Now, you don't need to pack up your bags and grow dreadlocks (no offence), but it's not a bad idea to cultivate a certain awareness of the things you could cut down on. By taking protective supplements and including certain foods in your diet you can reduce some of the effects of harmful oestrogen metabolites. And by choosing environmentally friendly goods and cleaning products we help the environment as well as ourselves.

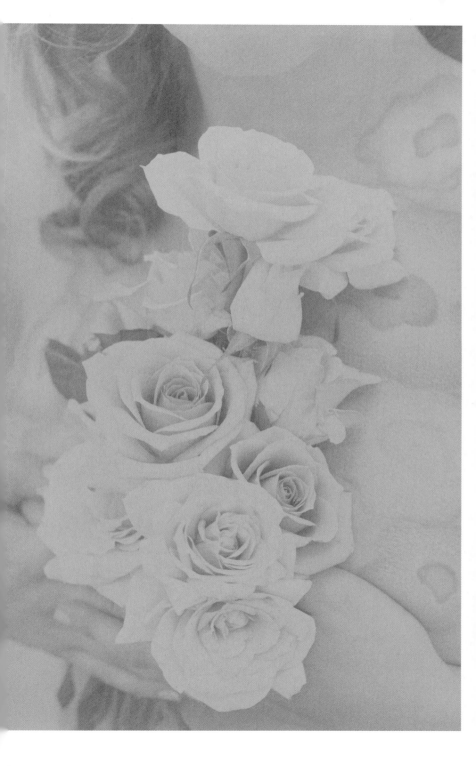

OESTROGENS

There are many natural substances that can help protect our breast tissue. Some of these substances block bad oestrogen, others provide an antioxidant (or baddy-quenching) effect.[140] Here are a few common examples.

Protective substances that help produce good oestrogen (2-hydroxyestrone)[141]	Substances that help produce bad oestrogen (16a-hydroxyestrone)[142]
Lignans found in plant fibre. Flax seed fibre is one of the richest sources of lignans.	**Plastic** containers and wrap can leach xeno-oestrogens into food and beverages.
Isoflavone herbs, e.g., red clover and kudzu.	**Chemicals,** e.g., insecticides, fungicides, pesticides (DDT, dieldrin), herbicides and organochlorines.
Umbelliferous herbs and vegetables including celery, fennel and parsley contain phyto-oestrogens. Fennel has confirmed oestrogenic action.	
	Adhesive glue on food packaging.
Phyto-oestrogens Other foods high in phyto-oestrogens include nuts, whole grains, apples and alfalfa.	**Insect repellent** and **hair products** that contain phthalates.
Nuts, seeds and legumes, e.g., alfalfa sprouts, sprouted legumes, fermented soy products.	**Detergents** that contain alkylphenols, amsonic acid, phenylphenols.
Seaweed Nori, Japanese seaweed and kelp.	**Drugs,** e.g., Diethylstilbestrol (DES), a synthetic oestrogen.
Indole-3-carbinol and sulforaphane is found in vegetables including broccoli, cauliflower, cabbage, Brussels sprouts and kale.	**Plastic additives,** e.g., bisphenol-A (BPA), polyvinyl chloride (PVC)
Omega 3 Fish oil and flax seed oil are rich sources of omega 3. Other sources include seafood, salmon, tuna, sardines and snapper.	**Gasoline additives,** e.g., benzene.
Green tea	

Store your drinking water in glass and heat food in the microwave using ceramic, glass or Pyrex dishware. This will help to reduce unwanted potentially harmful oestrogens that leach from plastics into the food.

Hormone replacement therapy[143]
ORAL CONTRACEPTIVE (OC)

Of course, it's up to you whether you choose to take the OC or not. Studies on it are conflicting. It's one of the best ways to stop pregnancy, but is thought to increase the risk of breast cancer. Thankfully, that risk lowers after 10 years of not taking the pill. The safest bet is to talk to your health care provider about the OC. If you decide it's for you, take a look at the option of the newer low-dose OCs available.

HRT

I (Lani) was instructed to take HRT for hormonal migraines and was told by a top gynaecologist that the risk of getting breast cancer while on HRT was very small. I have to tell you I wasn't tempted to follow up on my prescription because, as a naturopath, I know that herbs can have a wonderful effect on those nasty symptoms that occur when you have low oestrogen levels. Most women can take herbal formulas containing magnesium, sage, black cohosh, red clover, kudzu and dong quai, which work as well as HRT without the side effects. If you don't have breast cancer or a genetic link to breast cancer, try one of the formulas available from a health store or pharmacy. Most women find that it takes two weeks to three months to work (arghh). If it doesn't work, you may need an acidophilus and bifidus supplement. These beneficial bacteria help to convert the good oestrogen found in the herbs so they work in the body. If you are deficient in these goodies or have been taking antibiotics, the formula may not work as well or at all. You could also ask a naturopath to mix a specific formula for you.

The frustration I have with women taking herbal formulas for the first time is that, after buying one, they want it to work instantly. Then they go off the formula before it has had a chance to work, and try to live with hot flushes or go straight back on HRT. Other women feel cheated and switch it with another formula. It's important to highlight here that the herbal formulas are not an instant miracle cure – they can take up to three months to work.

If you do have breast cancer or a genetic link to breast cancer, or want to take HRT, there's a diagnostic test called the Oestrogen Metabolism Assessment which can be performed by the Great Smokies Diagnostic Laboratory (GSDL) in America to discover how you metabolise oestrogen. It's a simple urine analysis test that is performed twice over a period of time to make sure testing is accurate. Your naturopath can send a sample of urine to the GSDL. This will give you an idea as to whether you metabolise oestrogens into 'good' or 'bad' oestrogen metabolites. To simplify, a proper balance between good (2-hydroxyestrone) and bad (16a-hydroxyestrone) oestrogen metabolites is the key to good health. High levels of bad oestrogen metabolites are linked to breast cancer and other diseases, whereas good oestrogen metabolites may slow abnormal cell growth. Using this assessment, practitioners can monitor the physiological impact of flax seed (lignans), soy products (isoflavones), cruciferous vegetables (indole-3-carbinol) and other treatments (including natural or prescriptive hormone replacement therapy).[144]

After taking the metabolism assessment you should follow the dietary guidelines and advice in chapter five for reducing the risk of breast cancer. If your body has high levels of the bad metabolite, it's best to avoid soy and you should talk to a health professional about what to eat or supplement with to ensure a more balanced ratio. DIM is a wonderful supplement for normalising the way the body metabolises oestrogens, thus reducing high levels of bad oestrogen metabolites. Omega 3 fish oil, magnesium, B vitamins and zinc offer additional support. A vegetarian diet without soy is also known to help the body metabolise oestrogens beneficially and generally contains less fat, reducing the exposure to harmful oestrogens.

If you still want to take prescriptive HRT, talk to your specialist and then get a second opinion until you feel satisfied that you are fully informed. Ask to have a regular mammogram and follow other breast cancer reducing strategies. Avoid drinking alcohol; however, if you do choose to drink alcohol don't have more than two standard serves in one day while taking HRT, because this may increase your bad oestrogen metabolites.

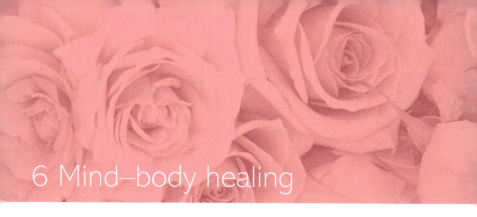

6 Mind–body healing

Psychoneuroimmunology

THE SCIENCE OF psychoneuroimmunology (PNI) is a relatively new field in medicine. It brings together knowledge from the study of endocrinology, immunology, psychology and neurology. Where once Western medicine focused solely on the body, PNI takes into account not just the body but how it interacts with the mind and the environment as well. Chinese and Indian medicines have long worked on the belief that the body and mind are not separate entities but are interwoven and one affects the other. Dr O Carl Simonton, a pioneer in psychosocial oncology, founder and medical director of the world-famous Simonton Cancer Centre in California, author of *Getting Well Again* and *The Healing Journey* and founder of PNI International (phew!!) believes that 'if medicine as we know it is to survive, it needs to become more flexible and embrace more aspects of the human being.'[145,146] There are various cancer centres around the world that follow this maxim with good results and it is becoming more commonly believed that PNI is another tool in the arsenal with which the medical world can fight cancer.

In his book *Taking Charge of Your Breast Cancer* Dr John Link talks of a woman he came to know who is termed a spiritual healer. Rosalyn Bruyere has the ability to see light and energy emitting from people's bodies. 'When she puts her hands close to me, I can feel a strange electrical sensation on the surface of my body below her hands,' he says. 'The incredible thing is that she is able to diagnose illness in different areas of the body with her senses.' Her ability is not 'pie in the sky' but has been scientifically verified at the UCLA Laboratory of Applied Kinesiology with Professor Valerie Hunt in 1978 and at the Menninger Clinic's Centre for Applied Psychophysiology in Topeka, Kansas, with Dr Elmer Green in 1994. 'My patients who have seen her describe a significant relief of pain and improved ability to tolerate treatment after experiencing her "running energy" with them,' says Dr Link. 'While I do not know how she does this I am convinced the effect is real. Physicians are asked to ignore perspectives on healing that are not quantifiable by traditional methods. I believe that cultivating openness to our patients' beliefs about healing is an integral part of patient care.'[147]

Dr Simonton is another specialist who believes in working with his patients' beliefs and is not opposed to visualisation and focused imagery. In his books he introduces the tools that lie at the heart of his programme: guided imagery and meditation techniques. The programmes he runs at his centre evolved from the concept that beliefs, feelings, attitudes and lifestyle are important factors affecting health. Both of these world-renowned experts recognise that you need to believe you can be proactive with your cancer. They say women who don't are less likely to pay attention to their diet, are more likely to suffer from depression, experience more pain and use more medication to alleviate it.

Let's explore some of the tools that you could use in addition to traditional remedies. None of the unorthodox methods we speak about in these pages are in any way meant to take over from traditional treatment, but if you believe in something use it. These techniques have sped and smoothed the healing process for many people. Many of them complement each other and several seem very similar, in fact a lot of the ancient techniques focus on keeping the body's life force or energy flowing unhindered. That might sound too spiritual or wacky for you but many so-called 'normal' people practise these techniques with good results. You don't have to sit around with your legs crossed saying 'ommmmm'. That's just a picture created for effect.

Many people like to pooh-pooh these practices but some well-known people have achieved amazing things through some of the techniques. Look at Louise Hay, who healed herself of cancer in six months, Brandon Bays, who healed herself of a tumour in six and a half weeks, and many sports and business people. Bear in mind that a lot of these methods have been evolving for many thousands of years. There will always be arguments against things that go against the common stream of thought, but you know what? Miracles happen around the world every day.

Laughter is the best medicine

Many years ago the well-known writer and editor Norman Cousins was diagnosed with a life-threatening disease. He cured himself by following a regime of high doses of vitamin C and belly laughing each day. What he started carried on with Hunter 'Patch' Adams, made famous by the film of the same name starring Robin Williams. Patch was on the brink of despair in 1969 when he committed himself to a psychiatric ward after a suicide attempt. While in the ward he saw first-hand the beneficial effects of his zany humour. He signed out of the psychiatric ward and enrolled in medical training. The real Patch wears a long grey ponytail, a thick, handlebar moustache, a silver fork earring in his ear and his eyes sparkle with mirth. He pushed the boundaries of the medical profession by living by the credence that joy should be a way of life. 'Not joke-for-jokes sake,' he says 'but to create an air of levity and humour.' It was a way of doing medicine that was inspiring, although it wasn't warmly received by the old school medical fraternity. Patch ignored the critics and went on to become famous for his clown noses and bee kisses.

'Happy, funny, loving, creative and co-operative; those were the requirements of my staff. With those qualities I knew great medicine would happen,' says Patch. 'And it did. It's extraordinary. If you don't concentrate on the pain, you don't feel it. Patients don't complain as much and the need for medication is reduced.' When he was about to be kicked out of medical school for 'excessive happiness' he could only recite what he knew to be true: '*The American Journal of Medicine* has found that laughter increases the secretion of endorphins and catecholamines which in turn increases oxygenation of the blood, relaxes the arteries, speeds up the heart and decreases blood pressure. This has a positive effect on all respiratory and cardiovascular ailments as well as increasing the immune system response overall.'[148]

Let's go back to endorphins. You've heard them mentioned in relation to exercise, I'm sure. Endorphins are defined as 'naturally occurring painkilling chemicals produced by the human nervous system that have qualities similar to opiate drugs'. They are believed to enhance the immune system, relieve pain, reduce stress, postpone the ageing process and some types can activate human NK (natural killer) cells which kill cancer cells.

Endorphins can be released by acupuncture, massage, chiropractic work, hydrotherapy, meditation, deep breathing, ribald laughter and even eating spicy food (yeah, go on, have that curry) and chocolate (hallelujah!). Exercise, particularly jogging, is another common endorphin releaser, the effects are commonly referred to as 'runner's high', which is why endorphin actions are often called 'inner jogging'.

In recognition of the positive effects of a good ol' giggle Yogic Laughter, which involves deep breathing and plenty of ha, ha, ha's, was originally introduced by Dr Madan Kataria in India. This has led to the formation of laughter clubs, clubs that celebrate the power of laughter. Pat Armitstead, a joyologist and founder of New Zealand's first laughter club, travelled through Russia with Patch Adams last year. She explains laughter exercises. 'The first part is fairly complex,' she says. 'You breathe in and go ho, ho, ho. The next part is even more complex, you breathe in and let out a ha, ha, ha. By then most people are smiling,' she says. These exercises raise heart and respiration rates, oxygenation of the system and reduce levels of stress.

At the Loma Linda University in California, Dr Lee Berk – associate director for the Centre for Neuroimmunology, assistant research professor at Loma Linda School of Medicine, and assistant clinical professor of health promotion and education in the School of Public Health – believes in the benefits of laughter so much he spends most of his time researching it.[149] Dr Berk believes that because a patient is more than just a disease, it's important to look at the whole person when providing medical treatment. His research has found that laughter decreases the levels of immunosuppressive hormones while boosting the levels of white blood cells that fight cancer tumours and support immunity. So while the last thing you might be feeling like doing right now is hamming it up, it might do you good to try. Your body doesn't know the difference between a sincere guffaw and a faked one.

Aromatherapy

Aromatherapy has proven to be beneficial in helping people going through breast cancer treatment. In fact it's a service offered in many cancer centres. However, there are cautions to take. The aromatherapy oils used must be of high quality and therein lies the problem. The untrained could confuse a $2 bargain bottle with the real thing. Don't take any risks. Get professional advice.

Aromatherapy involves the use of concentrated essential oils which come from grasses, flowers, leaves, fruit peel and woods. These oils are known to have therapeutic properties. They are used in massage, in bathing and by inhaling. Aromatherapy massage is useful for women with breast cancer because it helps with depression, pain and is very calming and nurturing.

Aromatherapy has proven to be helpful with:

- Depression
- Frustration
- Grief
- Hysteria
- Anxiety
- Insomnia
- Fear
- Hopelessness
- Panic attacks
- Sadness
- Worry
- Fatigue
- Nausea
- Enhancing wound healing

> Lemon or spearmint may help with nausea.

There are some oils that could be detrimental to someone undergoing breast cancer treatment so ensure you get expert advice. Mary Wakefield provides aromatherapy treatment at the Auckland Cancer Society. She is a trained radiotherapist and runs the Aromatherapy and Lymphoedema Clinic at Domain Lodge (see services and contacts at the back of the book for further details.) Call your local cancer society and they should be able to help you find someone reputable to speak with.

Acupuncture and acupressure

Acupuncture is a very old Chinese practice where very, very fine needles are applied to the surface of the body in strategic points. It works on the theory that there is an energy force running through the body known as Qi (pronounced Chee). When the pathways of this energy flow become obstructed or unbalanced this can cause illness. Practitioners choose their needle position based on the ailment. Acupressure is simply acupuncture without needles. Instead stimulation is applied to the area using pressure from the fingers or an instrument with a hard ball-shaped head. Acupuncture and acupressure raise levels of triglycerides, white blood cell counts and antibodies. The technique also stimulates endorphins and serotonin (feel-good hormone) levels.

Creative visualisation and affirmations

Shakti Gawain's book *Creative Visualisation* has been a bestseller for many years.[150] She says it's not necessary to believe in any metaphysical or spiritual ideas to have creative visualisation work for you. But you must have an open enough mind to try something new in a positive spirit. When you are ill you need to begin to picture yourself and affirm to yourself that you are in good health and see your illness as completely healed and cured. In the book Ms Gawain tells of the story of a man who wrote to her. He had been diagnosed with an inoperable brain tumour and the shock caused him to look deeply at his life and recognise where he was feeling stuck and frustrated. He used the techniques from the book (along with his regular medical care) to help him resolve some of his life issues. The tumour eventually disappeared and several years later had not returned. She says many people have told her that after they were diagnosed with terminal cancer they began using creative visualisation techniques. Years later, they are alive and healthy.[151] Who knows? We are not here to judge but to offer tools.

HOW TO CREATIVELY VISUALISE

To creatively visualise it's important to relax deeply. When your body and mind are deeply relaxed your brain wave pattern actually changes and becomes slower. This deeper, slower level is known as the alpha level (while your usual busy waking consciousness is called the beta level) and a lot of research is being done on its effects.

Some people find it extremely difficult to relax and just be. One trick is to close your eyes and go through each of your body parts and focus on relaxing them. Start from the scalp and move slowly downward to the forehead, eyes, cheeks, jaws, neck, shoulders, arms, hands, fingers, back, spine, chest, tummy, thighs, knees, calves, feet and toes. It's amazing how well it works.

OK, now that you're relaxed, think of yourself at a tranquil scene. This might be on the beach with the breeze flowing gently and the waves lapping on the shore or lying in a lush, green field with the birds singing in the air. Picture whatever you find soothing. Breathe deeply and rhythmically from the diaphragm. Deep breathing helps relax your muscles. If you can't actually 'see' the images don't worry you may not be a visual person. What you're after is the sense of calm and relaxation. The more you practise the easier it will become.

Now decide on what you want to work towards. Think of yourself as well and healed. Think in the present tense and include as many details as you can. Picture yourself as happy, healthy and relaxed. Now is also the time to introduce affirmations. According to Ms Gawain, affirmations are one of the most important elements to creative visualisation. To affirm means to make firm and an affirmation is a strong positive statement that something is already so.

Affirmations can be done silently, spoken aloud or written down. There are a few guidelines to the process of affirmations: always phrase affirmations in the present tense not in the future, for example 'I am now healthy' rather than 'I will be healthy'. And always phrase them in the most positive way you can, 'I am healthy and happy.' 'I am now relaxed, healthy and happy.' The shorter and more simple the statement the better. And try, as much you can, to believe what you're saying and put all of your energy into what you're saying. 'Every day in every way I am getting better and better.'[152]

The magic of touch

One of the most pampering things you can do for yourself at this time is to indulge in a facial. Not only are they great for your skin, they are also usually accompanied by a neck and shoulder massage. Some facials start with a foot massage and some will give you a foot massage or hand massage while your face mask is on. One of the rules in a good beauty therapist's training is to always have a hand on the client and never to leave them alone for too long. It's all about you and you need lots of that at this time.

The Touch Research Institute has found that massage therapy can reduce stress hormones, alleviate depressive symptoms, reduce pain and improve immune function.

Immediate massage therapy effects include reduced anxiety, depressed mood and anger and the longer-term effects include reduced depression and hostility, serotonin levels are raised and the number of natural killer cells and lymphocytes are increased (they're the cancer fighters).[153]

Meditation

Meditation is really a practice of taking time out for yourself and relaxing deeply. It is extremely calming and reduces blood pressure, chronic stress, anger and depression. Scientists have recently found that in addition to calming the nerves and reducing blood pressure, the regular practice of meditation as well as deep breathing can help the body produce endorphins. All the common bad feelings – anger, stress, etc. – induce the body to manufacture chemicals that can slow healing and shorten your lifespan, according to Candace B Pert in her book *Molecules of Emotion*.[154] Daily relaxation can help.

HOW TO MEDITATE

The best time of day to meditate is in the morning when your brain frequency is most likely at alpha (slow) but if you can't manage that don't get uptight about it – other times of the day can be effective too. You could try just before bed or just after lunch. Sit upright with your legs uncrossed, feet apart and flat on the floor, back straight, hands on your lap, head lowered and eyes closed. Start to focus on your breathing and, as much as possible, clear the mind. This becomes easier with time. You will still hear sounds around you, but they will not register on a conscious level. As you focus on your breathing, you should become deeply relaxed. Work down from your scalp to your toes to relax the body (see Creative visualisation on page 110). Your brain will now have slowed right down. You will probably find your mind wandering, this is very common, simply try to bring it back to focusing on your breathing. You can come out of a meditation by simply opening your eyes. Ideally you will meditate daily for 15 minutes. You may have noticed similarities with the process of creative visualisation and, yes, you can also use this time for goal setting and affirmations.

Reflexology

Reflexology is an ancient art of massage therapy that works on the feet. The interesting thing about the technique is that any congestion or tension in the foot is mirrored in a corresponding part of the body. Working on the area of the foot has proven beneficial effects on the injury or disorder in the correspondent body part. Another of the benefits of treatment seems to be an increase in ability to cope with the complexities of life on a physical, mental and emotional level. In a reflexology session the reflexologist applies pressure to the feet. A session takes about an hour and post-treatment people report a feeling of relaxation and wellbeing. The 1996 China Reflexology Symposium Report found foot reflexology to be 93.64% effective in treating 63 disorders.[155] On the reflexology chart, areas of the foot relating to the breast are on top of the foot, underarm lymph nodes on the ankle and lymph drainage in between the big toe and the second toe. When Karen was going through breast cancer treatment she had reflexology regularly and firmly believes this is why she didn't experience nausea or fatigue. Reflexology is common in Asian countries and you'll find reflexologists on every block. It's not so commonplace here, however, Brian Chen would like to see that changed. Brian owns Bliss – two reflexology specialist havens in Auckland. Brian brings all of his highly trained staff in from China, so they are trained in the home of the art. Even though there are only two Bliss locations open at present, plans are underway to set up more of the havens nationwide.

Reiki

There is some argument as to where Reiki (pronounced Ray-ke) originated from. Some say it is an ancient Japanese healing technique others say it is Tibetan. Wherever it hails from it is universally recognized for its ability to improve wellbeing. Rei means spiritually guided and Ki means life force or energy. Put together it means spiritually guided life force energy. Working on the same premise as acupuncture and acupressure, Ki represents the body's natural energy or life force. (Qi, Ki, the Chinese Chi, Sanskrit Prana and Ti or Ki in Hawaiian all stand for the same thing.) The theory goes that all living things have a life force flowing through them. If your life force is not flowing well or is at a low ebb, you will be susceptible to illness. The technique itself is a gentle 'hands-on' therapy in which the practitioner places her hands on or near different parts of your fully-clothed body. This might be the head, chest, abdomen or back. The aim is to get the life force energy flowing and balanced. Interestingly, in Canada recently, Dr Ahlam Manour of the College of Nursing received a $20,000 grant from the Canadian Breast Cancer Research Initiative to conduct a feasibility study of the effects of Reiki.[156] The study will investigate the effects of Reiki on anxiety levels, physical problems, spiritual wellbeing and blood counts in breast cancer patients undergoing chemotherapy.

Yoga

Yoga originally developed in India and has been around for over 5000 years. It is a highly respected form of exercise and experts say it helps prevent disease by keeping the life force energy flowing through the body. The practice involves a series of poses and deep-breathing that work something like self-massage. Some of the exercises are quite difficult but, with perseverance, the body will become more limber and supple and the exercises will become easier. It seems to be a general rule of thumb that the positions you find most uncomfortable are the best for you. Areas of weakness or decreased flexibility are said to be a trouble point in the energy system of the body. Mary says that yoga was the answer for her after having breast cancer surgery as it stretched out the scar tissue and made it more pliable so she didn't experience stiffness in the area. The many benefits that yoga is touted as having include helping with a number of physical complaints such as blood pressure, depression, chronic fatigue and stress. Yoga also improves strength and stamina, lowers fat and stimulates the immune system. There is also evidence to suggest yoga may be useful as complementary therapy to conventional medical treatment to help relieve symptoms associated with cancer.

TIPS FOR QUALITY SLEEP

1. Safely get regular exposure to daylight.
2. Avoid alcohol and caffeine in the evening, instead opt for a herbal drink with calming properties.
3. Wind down from a stimulating day by setting aside 'quiet time' to read and relax.
4. Don't doze on the sofa in front of the TV, go to bed when you begin to feel drowsy.
5. Reduce your light levels with dimmers or turn off bright lights before bedtime to create a relaxing environment.
6. Ensure your bedroom isn't too warm and that it is well ventilated.
7. Check your mattress is supporting your body.
8. Frustrated by not being able to fall asleep? Try deep-breathing techniques or get up and read until you feel sleepy.

Balance in life

One of the things most of us find difficult, whether unwell or in the peak of health, is balance. Let's face it, life today is busy and it's hard trying to find time for the family, for work, for me-time and for exercise and living well. In her book *Get A Life!*, lifecoach Andrea Malloy recommends setting goals, taking the best care of yourself and simplifying your daily life as much as you can. Don't look at this as the big picture – it's too hard! Just focus on trying to reduce areas of excessive busyness step-by-step over a period of time. 'As with any serious or chronic illness, breast cancer is certainly a catalyst for change, both in terms of a gaining a fresh perspective on life and prioritising what is really important to you,' says Malloy. 'But also, given the illness, there is an increased need to balance life with work and family and health, fitness and wellbeing.

This will be even more of a high priority than before.'

Like us, Malloy is a big advocate of self-care in finding balance and leaving stress at the door. The reality is you'll never escape some forms of this bugbear which is a hallmark of modern society and could well be a big contributor to illness. So don't be too hard on yourself, look after yourself by learning to say no to excessive demands, enrol in a yoga class, eat well and sleep well.

You are so beautiful

You know what it's like when you have a bout of the flu. Your nose is red from too much blowing, your eyes are watering and after a day on the couch you feel terrible and you don't look too fabulous either. But let's face it, you couldn't really give a hoot what you look like. The weird and wonderful thing is that if you got up and 'put your face on' you'd immediately feel better. Because you look good, you feel better. The same can be said of being ill with breast cancer. Obviously your top priority is getting well but looking at your makeup kit (or lack of it) could seriously help you get there. The lift you get from a bit of makeup impacts positively on your general wellbeing. In fact, beauty workshops specifically designed for women with cancer run throughout the country. They're called Look Good Feel Better and the name speaks for itself. Most women get the opportunity to register for a workshop at the hospital (if you don't, ask). And even the most hesitant and shy women who get themselves along to a session find it empowering. Some even find it life changing.

Nadine Powell, who runs the service, tells of one woman who'd been to Look Good Feel Better having never worn makeup in her life. 'And she's never had her lipstick off since,' smiles Powell. 'Some women think of it as frivolous or they feel they're not important enough. But these workshops are so important, we literally see people feel better and they tell us so with a smile on their faces.' The workshops address the unique making-up and grooming aspects that can come from having cancer treatment – dry skin, loss of eyebrows and eyelashes. The good news is these things are temporary. Yes! Post-treatment these things should return. But in the meantime there are a few tricks you can employ to minimise these changes. (That's the joy of makeup – it's all an illusion.) Clean skin and hair and light makeup that doesn't create a mask will make you feel much more confident. And when you look good you feel better.

One tip Nadine always gives to women who are experiencing hot flushes is to keep a spray bottle of toner or Evian water in the fridge and spray the feet regularly with it. 'That's the first pulse point so the freshness rises up the body,' she says. 'And if your eyes are sore or dry lie down and pop cold teabags or cucumber slices on them.'

HAIR

Hair or rather the loss of it through chemotherapy is one of the most traumatic things for many women who have undergone treatment for breast cancer. Some women say it's even worse than losing a breast because it's so visible. It's almost like an added insult to have your experience being tagged so visibly after all you've been through. To many of us our hair is our crowning glory. You only have to look at beauty statistics to see that's where most women spend their money. So it's very, very important to us. And if you're feeling distressed about the loss or possible loss of your hair you can take comfort in the fact that you're quite normal, any woman would be upset.

Hair follicles are filled with tiny blood vessels that make hair and cause it to grow. As we've already talked about, the cells in the body are constantly dividing and the cells in the area of the hair follicle are the third most active in the body. Chemotherapy targets healthy cells as well as cancer cells and it reaches the fastest growing cells first. That's why the drugs used during chemotherapy affect your hair and why hair is one of the first areas hit. 'The anti-mitotic drugs used in chemotherapy interfere with the cell division process and cause a narrowing and miniaturisation of the hair shaft,' says trichologist Nigel Russell of Holistic Hair. 'As a result one of two things may happen; the hair may fracture more easily and break off at the base or it may fail to form at all.' During treatment the hair follicle becomes distorted and oval in shape. 'If you look under a microscope at naturally curly hair you will find a similar shape, and if you explore the hair follicle it grows from it will be oval too. This is why you'll often find your hair will grow back curly after chemotherapy,' says Nigel. 'Usually this will last about eight to 12 months after treatment. The stress you are under while undergoing treatment is not to be underestimated in relation to hair growth/loss either. Physical and emotional stresses affect thyroid levels, growth hormone and blood sugar levels which can all have an adverse impact on the hair.'

The process of losing your hair may be gradual or dramatic. For some women only the hair on their head is affected, however, with others eyebrows, lashes and pubic hair can go too. Jo always complained that her legs and underarms didn't lose their hair, the only part she wouldn't have minded!

If you are undergoing chemotherapy and expect to lose your hair, many women suggest getting any length cut off before beginning treatment. That way if it starts to fall out it won't be so much of a shock. I saw one lovely lady at Look Good Feel Better a couple of years ago who had glorious waist length braids. She'd put her hair in braids before cutting them off and had sewn them into a hat. Even though the hat would never replace what she'd had before, it worked beautifully. And if you've never gone the short route this could be your chance to experiment. Some women look absolutely gorgeous with short hair and decide to keep it. Of course, if you hate it that's understandable.

Once you have finished treatment your hair should start growing back and after about two months you should have about an inch of hair. It may be a different colour (or you may be seeing your natural colour for the first time in years!) and as Nigel mentioned it may be curly. The hair on your head usually grows faster than eyebrows and eyelashes.

At a Look Good Feel Better workshop you'll get guidance on wigs, hats and turbans. But if once you've got a little growth happening you find you can't abide the short look, you could look at hair extensions. (I had a head injury many years ago and lost my hair. When it grew long enough I got extensions. I had to sit for nine hours and it cost hundreds of dollars but it was worth it! – Jenna.)

SKIN

When your body's being ravaged you can pretty much guarantee your skin will show some discord too – the two work closely together. Anaesthetic, radiotherapy, chemotherapy and other medications can all play havoc with your complexion. It will probably be extremely dry and sensitive and it may also look sallow and be flaking, patchy and red. The anatomy of breast cancer and the anatomy of skin are inextricably linked so what is great for your body will also be good for your skin. Dr Howard Murad, a world-renowned dermatologist from Los Angeles, who created the Murad Skincare Line and is the author of *Wrinkle Free Forever: The 5-Minute, 5-Week Dermatologists Program* was in New Zealand recently. The interesting thing he mentioned was that he'd had a couple of clients who had breast cancer and he discovered that when they followed his programme for their skin, which is based on healthy living principles and includes lots of supplements and water, they also experienced improvement in other areas such as lymphoedema and fatigue.[157] Food for thought...

What you can do
You need to find the most gentle, natural cleansers and moisturisers you can find.
- Using a gentle cleanser and a sponge (the $2 shop has these) use tepid water to cleanse the skin. Do this morning and night.
- When choosing your moisturiser opt for a soft, sensitive skin formulation that's loaded with antioxidants and vitamins and that makes your skin feel smooth, soft and supple. (Skip any special treatment creams at this time.) Massage it into your face blending it down onto your neck and across your décolleté too. (Many people forget this step.) You can get a fabulous natural skin nourisher by cracking open a vitamin E capsule or using rosehip oil.
- Protect: use a sunscreen, perhaps your moisturiser may include a broad spectrum sunscreen but you need something that protects you from both UVA and UVB rays. (Try to avoid chemical-based ones if you can.)

BODY SKIN

It probably won't be just your facial skin that's experiencing difficulties at this time. Follow the same suggestions for your body as we've used for the face. Sharon Osbourne and some of the celebrity guests she has on her television show swear by Bertoli light olive oil. They say it absorbs well and gives you silky soft skin. (All natural and we like that right now.) Note: If you can't find it at your local supermarket try specialist Italian grocery stores or delicatessens – or ask your local supermarket to stock it!

It's important you build up your skin's resistance, hydration and resilience levels in every way you can. There are several ways you can achieve this (and many of these things you'll already be doing for your general wellbeing anyway):
- Eat loads of fresh fruit and vegetables – antioxidants are the key to fighting free radicals (which are like villains).
- Drink pure, spring water and fresh juice – your skin will love the goodness.

- Use pure high lignan flax seed oil as a dressing over salads. (See page 86.)
- Look for pure, organic skincare products. The jury's still out on controversial parabens and other common skincare ingredients and you want to be very careful with yourself at this stage. Parabens are widely used as preservatives in skincare (as well as in food, pharmaceutical preparations and some household products). Another ingredient under the microscope is sodium laurel sulphate (SLS). The problem is both of these ingredients have been touted as oestrogen mimics; however, the general school of thought is that there is a lack of quantitative data on any of these findings. What is known is that the body can absorb them and if they do have the oestrogen-mimicking abilities suspected, they could potentially create hormonal havoc in your body and that's the last thing you need right now. It's like so many things to do with cancer, nobody knows for sure. But if you're looking for à la natural (because many naturals aren't actually truly natural) A'Kin, Dr Hauschka, Living Nature, Simplicité, Skinfood and Trilogy were all created on these principles. David Lyons, the man who created Simplicité, actually started his career in the cancer ward of the Royal Brisbane Hospital.

Supplementation

Crash dieting, alcohol, overexposure to the sun and pollutants, smoking and stress can all adversely affect the beauty of your hair, skin and nails. Check your diet to be sure you are getting enough protein, and that you are drinking lots of liquid. Don't be overzealous on cutting back on fats since certain fatty acids are important for healthy skin and shiny hair.

- **Moisturisers** with vitamin A, C and E have the ability to increase skin elasticity and decrease skin roughness.
- **Increase circulation** with ginger and turmeric. Add these to your foods or choose a supplement form. Your nails, skin and hair all require good blood circulation to bring them the nutrients they need and to take away the waste products they produce.
- **Good oils** such as evening primrose, flax seed and/or fish oil help keep your skin, hair and nails in wonderful condition…oil your body from within.
- **Marine collagen and lyophilised marine protein** help provide the body with ingredients to regenerate the skin matrix in damaged ageing skin.

- **Antioxidants** help prevent free radical damage to the skin, premature ageing, fine lines and wrinkles. Take potent antioxidants such as ProenOthera, grapeseed, pinebark and green tea.
- **Herbs** for skin and clear complexions include red clover, burdock, echinacea, dandelion root and milk thistle.
- **Premature greying hair** Naturopaths have reported success with a high-protein diet plus two tablespoons each of brewer's yeast and flax seed oil daily, and B-complex, choline, PABA and copper supplements.
- **Hair growth** Use stimulating oils and herbs such as rosemary, grapeseed, apple extract and horse chestnut extract or oil treatments with jojoba or almond oil. Nutritional support from spirulina, chlorophyll and aloe vera juice may be helpful.
- **Splitting and weak hair and nails** Take tissue salt combination U (homeopathic mineral) along with a calcium/magnesium supplement and lyophilised marine protein with EPO and zinc.

MAKEUP: WHY BOTHER?

Because it will make you look and feel so much better and help increase your confidence. If you've never been a makeup kind of girl you might find Look Good Feel Better changes your ways forever. One girl I know (she was 30 at the time) always eschewed makeup until attending a workshop. Now she's sold. Makeup can up your self-esteem and make you feel better even when you feel really bad. Some people worry they don't know how to use it but believe us, basic makeup is not so hard to do. The most important thing here is you and feeling good. Do what feels right – you're not setting out to be a makeup artist after all.

If you can't afford the entire list, leave some out. Concentrate on the areas that concern you most. If

> What you will need:
> - Foundation or tinted moisturiser
> - Concealer
> - Bronzer or loose, translucent powder
> - Eyebrow makeup or pencil (if you opt for a pencil, look for one that glides on smoothly and easily, test it on your hand). Try not to choose very dark shades.
> - Eyeshadow (a couple of neutral shades is fine)
> - Mascara
> - Blusher
> - Lipgloss or lipstick
> - A set of makeup brushes will be useful
> - Cotton buds
> - A mirror will help too!

blotchy skin and/or dark circles are your bugbears spend your cash on foundation – we can double up on foundation and concealer. Eyeshadow can double as eyebrow makeup or you could forgo the eyeshadow and just use an eyebrow pencil. If your eyelashes haven't come back yet forgo the mascara. If you've got bronzer, leave out the blusher – the bronzer can do double duty. But the lippy is, I think, essential. Lipstick/gloss can light up a face instantly. Are you ready? To the mirror, madame!

Base: Your skin will be moisturised and sun protected from your skincare regime so foundation is your first step. Use your sponge, brush or your fingers – whatever you feel comfortable with. Either apply the foundation to the top of your hand and dab or dot from there – forehead, cheeks, nose and chin. And then spread. Ensure you blend. You don't have to be an expert just blend in any lines.

Concealer: If you're using concealer or foundation, get the concealer brush (it will be a flat-ended shape) or use your fingers and dab under the eye area at any dark circles. You should experience an instant lift. Many people don't use foundation but just use concealer on any areas of the face they need to lift or cover.

Powder/bronzer: If you're using powder or a bronzer, get a big, fat, fluffy brush and sweep it every-so-lightly over the face. You don't want overkill here just a very light veil to 'set' your makeup.

Eyebrows: Often underutilised, the eyebrows act as a fabulous frame for the face. Often if you've been through chemotherapy your eyebrows will either be sparse or not there at all and even if you're not a makeup aficionado you could well feel naked without them. But never fear there are ways to combat this. What you're looking to achieve is a fine arch.

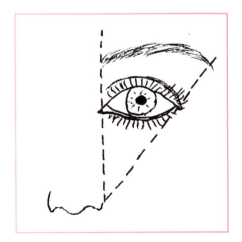

Using your eyebrow pencil (or a ruler) as a guide, run it in a straight line from the side of your nostril to above the eye. This is where your eyebrow should start. Then take the pencil again and run it in a straight line from outer corner of the eye and mark where the pencil ends at eyebrow height. This is where you want your brow to end. Then ever-so-carefully pencil in tiny, light strokes to fill in the shape. You should still be able to see where your brow was even if all the hair has gone. Using a brow brush go softly over the line with an eyeshadow to soften any harsh edges. Transformed!!

Eyeshadow: If you're using eyeshadow sweep a creamy or neutral colour over the entire eyelid. If you wish to create accent and make the eyes stand out, use a darker colour in the outer corner of the eyelid in the shape of a 'v' on its side (<). Take the darker colour in the eye socket crease to about the same length as the pupil and do the same along the line close to the upper eyelashes. Blend, blend, blend – that's the biggest trick.

Eyeliner: Using your eyebrow pencil or an eyeliner pencil – try not to use black it's a bit harsh, use a light or dark brown or even a pretty colour if you're feeling adventurous – draw a line along the eye close to the top lashes from the outer corner to the inner corner. Now use your pencil to draw a line under the eye as close to the lashes as you can. Work from the outer corner to about mid or three quarters of the way along. Using a sponge tipped applicator go over the line with eyeshadow to soften it (a cotton bud will do). Blend. That may sound like parroting but the key with all makeup is to blend any lines so it's kind-of blurred. Harsh lines are extremely unflattering. This is really important if your lashes are gone as eyeliner can create the illusion of a frame for the eyes.

Mascara: If you're using mascara, coat lashes from the lash line to the ends. If they're sparse, investing in a product like Origins Underwear for Lashes or one of the mascaras with a primer one end and mascara the other will help thicken them. L'Oréal, Maybelline and Revlon all do one. The primer helps thicken individual lashes and makes them longer which will create the illusion that there are more of them.

Blusher: An ever-so-light sweep of blush or bronzer on the apples of the cheeks swept back to the hairline will add an indefinable glow.

Lips: The *pièce de résistance* is the lips. If you've chosen to get a lip pencil, outline the lips with it. A trick of the trade is to use it to fill the lips in too; it will help your lipstick to last longer. If you've chosen a lipstick, apply with a brush or, if you can't be bothered with that entire hullabaloo, simply apply it straight from the lipstick container. If you want a really modern look, just swipe some gloss on and reapply it regularly.

6 | MIND–BODY HEALING

HANDS AND FEET

Most people don't realise that the finger and toe nails are one of the first places to show tell-tale signs of illness. So if you're going through cancer chances are they will be showing a bit of wear and tear. You may see a line or multiple lines in the nails after chemotherapy. You could also see pigmentation, discolouration and the nails may be more dry and brittle than usual. They may even be lifting up from the nail bed. But never fear there are things you can do that will help.

One of the best things for nails is to soak them in warm olive oil (that Bertoli has its uses yet again!). The nails seem to drink up the nourishment. If you're having problems with breakages or ripping try to resist the urge to just tear them off, cut them off instead. They'll be better for it and you probably will too. By ripping off nails you run the risk of pulling them off low past what is commonly called the 'quick' (but in scientific terms is called the hyponychium). This area is rich with nerve endings so you'll end up tender. A lovely thing you can do for you is to give yourself a basic manicure and pedicure. Or direct someone else to do it or, even better, book in at a beauty therapist where you'll get a massage as well.

Manicure: If you've already got some sort of nail coating on remove it with the nail polish remover and a cotton ball. Next lightly file nails into shape. Use the file in one direction – using a see-saw motion isn't good for the nails. Just shape the top of the nail you don't want to file the sides away. If you do this it will weaken the nail. Soak the nails in the warm water or oil if desired. If you're applying cuticle cream take the hands out one by one, dry them off with a hand towel or paper towel

---

What you'll need for a basic manicure and/or pedicure:
- Clippers or nail scissors
- File (not steel)
- Three-way buffer

Optional:
- Cuticle cream
- Base coat or strengthener
- Top coat
- Nail polish
- Non-acetone nail polish remover (it's gentler than acetone)
- Cotton wool balls
- Cotton buds or orangewood stick
- Bowl of warm water or olive oil
- Hand towel
- Paper towel
- Footbath

and massage the cream into the fingertips. Opening a vitamin E oil capsule will also work well here. Using the cotton bud or orangewood stick (wrapped with cotton wool at the end) gently push back the cuticles. Soak in warm water, dry off. You could use the polish remover and cotton wool ball here again to remove any residue that may hinder your nail paint's adherence. Paint with basecoat or strengthener. If you're using colour, apply two coats after this. Wait 20 minutes and finish off with top coat.

Pedicure: Soak feet in lavender scented water. If you're lucky enough to have a foot spa turn it on and rest there for a while. Toenails tend to be quite tough so this will soften them. Take feet out one by one and dry off. Cut the toenails straight across with the clippers or nail scissors. If necessary file for a smooth finish. As for fingers massage in cuticle cream or vitamin E oil and gently push back cuticles. Soak excess off (you could again use nail polish remover here to aid adherence) and paint.

Note: If you're due for any sort of surgery leave out the nail colour. The anaesthetists like to be able to see the colour of your nail beds.

WHAT TO WEAR

If you don't choose to have breast reconstruction, and many people don't, you'll probably be wearing a prosthesis. Many specialist lingerie shops offer an excellent variety of prostheses and cleverly adapted prosthesis pockets fitted into underclothing and swimsuits. (Your local Cancer Society should be able to point you in the right direction here.) Prostheses are also known as breast forms and they come in soft, flesh coloured silicon shapes designed to mimic the shape and weight of the breast. They come in all shapes, weights and sizes and most come with a nipple but if it's not nipple enough for you, you can buy a stick on version. There's more to wearing a breast form than aesthetic reasons, losing a breast can alter your balance and, if it's not evened out, you could be up for back or neck pain or even spinal curvature. The good news is there is a government benefit to help pay for them. Ask your doctor.

If you're sensitive from surgery or radiation therapy you'll be choosing a bra without underwires. Sports crop tops are the most comfortable as they don't have any 'diggy in' bits. You'll probably also be looking for finer quality fabrics in your tops and t-shirts now too. Soft cottons and fine silks feel comfortable on the skin. Polar fleece can be very comforting too.

Some pretty lacy lingerie could be just what you're looking for if you're feeling a bit battered after your experience. Spoil yourself and make yourself feel lovely.

A note to friends and family

One of the nicest things you could do for your loved one is to give them a beauty therapy voucher. Just ensure, if you don't know the clinic you're buying the voucher from, that you talk to them first. If they come across as warm, friendly and nurturing you've got the right place. Also make sure it's not too noisy – look for a haven of tranquillity. Let the clinic know that the voucher is being bought for someone who is going through cancer treatment as certain treatments and aromatherapy oils (and many clinics burn them throughout the day) can be detrimental.

Other things you could do for her include:
- **Arrange a pretty vase of flowers:** It's a simple pick-me-up but it works a treat.
- **Bills:** Make sure all of her bills are up-to-date. These are the kinds of things that go on the back burner in times of distraction.
- **Cleaning:** Just simple things like vacuuming, clothes washing, etc.
- **Cook her a meal:** What a treat it is when someone else cooks and it always tastes so much better!!
- **Do the gardening:** Not all of us have the luxury of having a gardener and those weeds can grow quickly.
- **Drive her to appointments:** This can be a real bind when you're undergoing treatment. A friendly driver can take the load off.
- **Fill up her freezer with heat-and-eat meals:** It's incredible how helpful this is to someone who's unwell.
- **Give her a funny card:** As you can see in the chapter on laughter that's like giving her a tonic!
- **Hire your friend a housekeeper:** Ahhh, now here's a good one. There's nothing nicer than having the little fairies in the house. It's magic. Somehow an unclean house makes you feel bad.
- **Listen if she wants to talk:** This seems so simple but many people don't specialise in listening.
- **Look after the children:** It's terribly hard trying to be a mother when you're experiencing a serious illness. Having someone trustworthy looking after the children is a treat.

- **Make sure there's a detachable showerhead to make showering easier:** Showers can be awkward when your body is under strain, versatility is very helpful.
- **Organise a weekend away full of laughter:** Another fun tonic – a change of scene can be refreshing.
- **Pampering:** Give her a home facial. Use yummy ingredients from the fridge and pantry. Banana, honey, egg, soaked desiccated coconut, avocado and mango are a few fragrant ideas for a face mask. Take her to the hairdresser to have her head massaged and hair washed, dried and styled.

> BUT THE MOST IMPORTANT THING IS TO JUST BE THERE, SUPPORTIVE AND TRUE.

- **Reflexology:** Book her in for some reflexology.
- **Shopping:** Get the groceries for her and her family or do it together online.

AND DON'T FORGET: SUPPORT THE SUPPORT

When someone you love has breast cancer you face your own challenges. There will be times when you will need support too, so don't be afraid to reach out. You will feel better if you have a chance to vent and come to terms with your feelings. Use some of the techniques we talk about in Chapters five and six. These techniques are for everyone, not just for those with chronic illness. They're stress-busters. In fact every single person on this planet would probably find utilising some of those techniques beneficial.

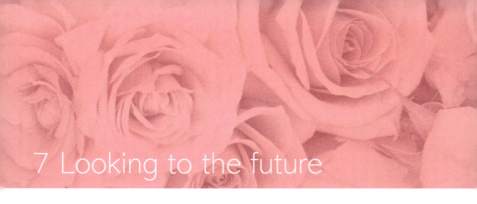

7 Looking to the future

Can we prevent breast cancer?

THE RESEARCH GOING ON around the world into breast cancer is phenomenal. And people from all walks of life – big business and the girl next door – are getting behind the cause to raise funds for research and raise awareness. This is a wonderful thing because it's these loud voices and the power of the people that will make the difference in our quest for answers. We need those answers because the information we have right now is not nearly enough. For instance, if you take a look at the wide cross-section of people who get breast cancer it would seem that following 'the rules' by keeping weight down, not drinking too much alcohol, eating a sensible diet, exercising regularly and having babies earlier means you won't get breast cancer, right? Yeah right! There is no life on Mars yet either. As we mentioned earlier there are women who follow 'the rules' who still get breast cancer and women who break every rule in the book who don't.

Lowering oestrogen levels in the body would seem to be crucial. Exercising regularly is also crucial. Avoiding highly processed foods also seems to be a strong contender in the prevention of breast cancer. But we quite simply don't yet know exactly how we might prevent breast cancer. Mr Trevor Smith, breast specialist at Ascot Hospital in Auckland believes breast cancer gets treated out of context of general health. 'You need to look at your overall health. If I see a woman who is obese and smoking coming in to have a mammogram that's very good but she's more at risk of heart disease, diabetes, and/or lung disease than she is of breast cancer,' he says. 'It's like living dangerously and wearing a parachute. Health and disease is all about the nuts and bolts of the things that occur over the years. The Alison Roe Run to Heal event for breast cancer makes sense. If everybody did events like that and exercised regularly we'd probably see people going off their antidepressant medication, hypertensive medication and diabetic medication as well.' Indeed, increasing numbers of women survive breast cancer and end up dying of an unrelated cause. Heart disease kills far more women in the world than breast cancer. Long Island's Coldspring Harbour Laboratory, where cancer research is a huge part of the day, predicts cancer will be a managed disease by 2015. That means controlled rather like we've controlled tuberculosis and pneumonia. So we're making progress. Dr Susan Love believes we will soon be able to individually tailor treatment to the type of breast cancer a woman has. 'The beginning of this is happening and it's very exciting,' she says. 'I'm convinced getting to where the breast cancer starts is how we're going to eradicate it. It's time to get rid of it because it's been around for far too long. There are diseases and cancers we can cure and prevent now and we need to do that with breast cancer.'

A positive conclusion

Once your initial treatment is over you may find well-meaning friends saying to you 'great, now that's over you can get on with your life.' What they don't understand is that, in some ways, your life will never be the same again. You will be well and happy again, but in many ways you'll be different. It will take time to come to terms with what you've been through. Deep down you will more than likely feel nervous that your breast cancer will come back.

After treatment is over many people experience a down-time – they've been fighting for so long they don't quite know what to do now the battle is over. As Dr Marisa Weiss explains: 'Instead of feeling ready to get on with your life, you feel lost, kind of nowhere, fearful that the cancer might grow back because you're no longer doing anything active to keep it away. You might even start worrying whether the treatment you had really worked. What you need is time, time to catch your breath, to figure out where you are in your life. And the further out you are from treatment, the more time "under your belt", the better you'll feel.'[158] Take a look at your life and figure out where you want to go from here. Many women report they take better care of themselves after breast cancer and most women return to lives as full as, and often richer personally, than they had before their illness. 'One positive thing about surviving cancer is that you really do appreciate what you have, how precious life is and how precious the time you have is, and you don't let the little things bother you anymore,' says Helen. Enjoy your life, your loved ones and your art, writing, cooking, reading or whatever it is you adore doing. You'll probably find you'll not put off until tomorrow the things on your wish list like you might have done in the past. Barbara Delinsky, well-known author of *Coast Road, Through My Eyes* and *Uplift* bought herself a sports car after her breast cancer treatment was over. And why not?

She deserved it. And you deserve to spoil yourself too. OK, granted, you might not be a bestselling author with the disposable funds to buy a new car but you get the picture. You have walked a tremendous journey and have experienced the terror and the blessings that come with a serious illness. You will probably still have good days and bad days, days when you lament what you've lost, days when you feel fear at the slightest ache or bump in your body. Once treatment is over you will find yourself back on the path of your life albeit having faced your own mortality and with a psyche and a body that has changed in some ways. Only you can decide the role that having had breast cancer will play in your life but we hope you live in hope and happiness. And please remember, you will never walk alone...

Services and contacts

Getting a second opinion
Genetic testing for breast cancer and counselling can be performed in:
- **Auckland** at Northern Regional Genetic Services, lower ground floor, Auckland Public Hospital.
- **Wellington** (covering the geographic area from Gisborne and Taranaki to Nelson) at Central Regional Genetic Services, Private Bag, Wellington Hospital.
- **Christchurch** at Southern Regional Genetic Services, Hagley Hostel, Christchurch Hospital.

New Zealand breast cancer organisations and other useful contacts

Aromatherapy and Lymphoedema Clinic
Contact Mary Wakefield
Appointments can be made through the Auckland Cancer Society's Support Services (see below)

Breastscreen Aotearoa
Phone 0800 270 200

Breast Cancer Research Trust
Phone 0800 BCRT CURE (0800 2278 2873)

Breast Cancer Network
Provides a survivor network
Phone (09) 526 8853

Breast Cancer Support Services
Phone (09) 526 8853

Busting With Life Dragon Boat Team
Phone 0800 800 426

Cancer Information Service
Phone 0800 800 426

Cancer Society of New Zealand Inc
National Office
PO Box 12145, Wellington
Phone (04) 494 7270

Auckland Division
PO Box 1724, Auckland
Phone (09) 308 0160

Waikato/Bay of Plenty Division
PO Box 134, Hamilton
Phone (07) 838 2027

Central Districts Division
(Covers: Taranaki, Wanganui,

Manawatu, Hawke's Bay
and Gisborne)
PO Box 5096, Palmerston North
Phone (06) 364 8989

Wellington Division
(Covers: Marlborough, Nelson,
Wairarapa and Wellington)
52 Riddiford Street, Wellington
Phone (04) 389 8421

Canterbury/West Coast Division
PO Box 13450, Christchurch
Phone (03) 379 5835

Otago/Southland Division
PO Box 6258, Dunedin
Phone (03) 477 7447

Fertility Associates
Richard Fisher
Phone: (09) 520 9520 or
www.fertilityassociates.co.nz

Look Good Feel Better
Phone (09) 308 0245

**Lymphoedema
Support Network**
Phone 0800 800 246 or
(09) 308 0162

**The New Zealand
Breast Cancer Foundation**
0800 902 732

**The New Zealand Foundation
for Cosmetic Plastic Surgery**
0800 266 552

**The New Zealand Medical
Council**
(04) 384 7635

**Waikato Breast Cancer
Research Trust**
Phone (07) 834 3665

Well Women's Nursing Service
Phone (09) 523 0263

Women's Health Action
Phone (09) 520 5295

Further reading to help you through

A Cancer Battle Plan by Anne E Frahm & David J Frahm (Putnam Publishing Group, new edition 1998).

A Short, Short Guide to a Happy Life by Anna Quindlen (Random House, 2000).

A Woman's Decision: breast care, treatment and reconstruction by K Berber & J Bostwick III (Quality Publishing, 1994).

Anatomy of an Illness as Perceived by the Patient by Norman Cousins (Bantam, 1991).

Beating Our Breasts compiled by Margaret Clark (Cape Catley, 2000).

Creative Visualization by Shakti Gawain (Bantam, 1983).

Dr Susan Love's Breast Book III by Susan M Love MD with Karen Lindsey (Perseus Publishing, 2000).

Everyone's Guide to Cancer Therapy: how cancer is diagnosed, treated and managed day to day by M Dollinger, E Rosenbaum & G Cable (Somerville House Books Ltd, 1994).

Ice Bound by Dr Jerri Nielsen (Miramax Books, 2001).

Intimacy: Living As A Woman After Cancer by Jacquelyn Johnson (NC Press, 1987).

It's Not About The Bike by Lance Armstrong (Penguin, 2000).

Living Beyond Breast Cancer by Marisa C Weiss & Ellen Weiss (Three Rivers Press, 1998).

Living Beyond Limits by David Spiegel (Ballantine Books, 1994).

No Less A Woman: Femininity, Sexuality & Breast Cancer by Deborah Hobler Kahane. *Sexuality and Fertility After Cancer* by Leslie R Schover (Wiley, 1997).

Reflections on Healing and Regeneration by Martin Seligman (Chronicle Books, 2004).

Spirited Women – Journeys with Breast Cancer by Petrea King (Random House, 1995).

Take Charge of Your Breast Cancer by Dr John S Link (Henry Holt, 2002).

The Breast Cancer Survival Manual by Dr John S Link (Henry Holt, 2000).

The Unremarkable Nipple by Sue McLeod (Dunmore Press, 1998).

There's More To Life than My Right Breast by Cyndi Kaplan-Freiman (New Holland Publishers, 2002).

Unbreakable Spirit: facing the challenge of cancer in New Zealand by Karen McMillan (Tandem Press, 2003).

Uplift: practical and reassuring advice from breast cancer survivors by Barbara Delinsky (Piatkus Books, 2002)

Welcome To The Amazon Club by Jane Bissell (Longacre Press, 2004).

Women of Silence, The Emotional Healing of Breast Cancer by Grace Adamson (2nd edition, 2003).

You Can Conquer Cancer by Ian Gawler (Hill of Content Pub Co, 1984).

You Can Get Through This! How to stay positive when you're coping with breast cancer by Domini Stuart (Domini Stuart, 2001).

Your Life in Your Hands by Professor Jane Plant (Virgin Publishing Ltd, 2001).

Useful websites

American Cancer Society Breast Cancer Network: www.cancer.org

Bliss Reflexology
www.blissreflexology.com

Breast Cancer Network New Zealand Inc. An NZ-wide grassroots organisation for women with breast cancer and their supporters:
www.breastcancer.nz.co.net

Breast Link Medical Group: www.breastlink.com

www.breastcancer.org

Cancer Information Service: www.cancernz.org.nz

Cancer Research UK: www.cancerresearchuk.org

Coping with Cancer magazine: www.copingmag.com

Dr Susan Love's website: www.susanlovemd.com

PubMed Central (PMC) is the U.S. National Institutes of Health (NIH) free digital archive of biomedical and life sciences journal literature: www.ncbi.nlm.nih.gov/entrez/query.fcgi

The Breast Cancer Research Trust: www.bcrt.co.nz

The New Zealand Breast Cancer Foundation: www.nzbcf.org.nz

The Royal New Zealand College of general practitioners:
www.rnzcgp.org.nz/breast.php

Other websites that may be of interest

www.facingourrisk.org

www.hopkinsmedicine.org

www.livingwithit.org/breast

www.livingbeyondbreastcancer.org

www.mdanderson.org

www.menagainstbreastcancer.org

www.youngsurvival.org

www.groups.yahoo.com/group/bosombuds

www.health.yahoo.com/health/centers/breast_cancer

www.oncology.com

www.oncolink.upem.edu

www.med.standord.edu/healthlibrary

www.nccn.org

www.breastcancer.net

www.med.jhu.edu/breastcancer/artemis

www.beans.org

www.cancerandcareers.org

www.breastcancerinfo.com

www.simontoncenter.com

Endnotes

1. S.M. Love, MD, with K. Lindsey, *Dr Susan Love's Breast Book*, 3rd Edn, (Cambridge, MA: Perseus Publishing, 2000) pp (1):5–6.
2. ibid pp (2):25–32.
3. M. Stoppard, *Woman's Body,* (London: Dorling Kindersley Ltd, 1991) p (9):66
4. N.K. Horner and J.W. Lampe, "Potential mechanisms of diet therapy for fibrocystic breast conditions show inadequate evidence of effectiveness", *J Am Diet Assoc.* 2000 Nov;100(11):1368–80.
5. L. Oveson, "Vitamin therapy in the absence of obvious deficiency. What is the evidence?", *Drugs.* 1984 Feb;27(2):148–70.
6. E.R. Gonzalez, "Vitamin E relieves most cystic breast disease; may alter lipids, hormones", *JAMA.* 1980 Sep 5;244(10):1077–8.
7. G.S. Sundaram et al., "alpha-Tocopherol and serum lipoproteins", *Lipids.* 1981 Apr;16(4):223–7.
8. R.S. London et al., "Evaluation and treatment of breast symptoms in patients with the premenstrual syndrome", *J Reprod Med.* 1983 Aug;28(8):503–8.
9. R.J. Barth et al., "Detection of Breast Cancer and Screening Mammography Allows Patients to be Treated with Less-Toxic Therapy", *Am J Roent.* 184 (2005): 324–329.
10. *Breast test fears drop with medication*. Retrieved 19 Jan 2005 from http://www.breastcancersource.com
11. *Understanding your risk*. Retrieved 24 Mar 2005 from "The New Zealand Breast Cancer Foundation" http://www.nzbcf.org.nz/frame.htm
12. I. Wolf et al., "Diabetes mellitus and breast cancer", *Lancet Oncol.* 2005 Feb;6(2):103–11.
13. A. Nkondjock and P. Ghadirian, "Risk factors and risk reduction of breast cancer", *Med Sci* (Paris). 2005 Feb;21(2):175–180.
14. J. Blue et al., "Overview of breast cancer prevention – a search for the causes of breast cancer", *NZ GP Mag.* 7 Oct 1998. 32–35.
15. Wolf et al., loc. sit.
16. Nkondjock and Ghadirian, loc. sit.
17. The Royal New Zealand College of General Practitioners, *Early detection of breast cancer*. Retrieved 16 Feb 2005 from http://www.rnzcgp.org.nz/breast.php
18. *Breast cancer facts* (1 Oct 2003). Retrieved 16 Feb 2005 from "The New Zealand Breast Cancer Foundation" http://www.nzbcf.org.nz/news/display.asp?itemId=190
19. C.M.M Lawes et al., "The epidemiology of breast cancer in Pacific women in New Zealand", *NZ Med J.* 1999;112:354–7.
20. A.E. Lethaby et al., "Age and ethnicity as prognostic factors influencing overall survival in breast cancer patients in the Auckland region: Auckland Breast Cancer Study Group", *NZ Med J.* 1992;105:485–8.
21. E. Deligeoroglou et al., "Oral contraceptives and reproductive system cancer", *Ann N Y Acad Sci.* 2003 Nov;997:199–208
22. D.R. Mishell Jr., "Expanded role for OCs. Question and answer", *Dialogues Contracept.* 1994 Summer;4(3):8.

23. R. Chandran, "Contraception and the big 'C'", *Malays J Reprod Health* 1992 Jun;10(1):1–5.
24. H.B. Peterson and P.A. Wingo, "Oral contraceptives and breast cancer: any relationship?", *Contemp Oncol.* 1992 Dec;2(10):13–14, 19–20, 2.
25. International Planned Parenthood Federation IPPF and International Medical Advisory Panel IMAP, "IMAP statement on Norplant subdermal contraceptive implant system", *IPPF Med Bull* 1993 Apr;27(2):1–3.
26. A.Z. Bluming, "Hormone replacement therapy: the debate should continue", *Geriatrics.* 2004 Nov;59(11):30–1, 35–7.
27. S.M. Harman et al., "Is the WHI relevant to HRT started in the perimenopause?", *Endocrine.* 2004 Aug;24(3):195–202.
28. M.A. Richards et al., "Influence of delay on survival in patients with breast cancer: a systematic review", *Lancet.* 1999;353:1119–26.
29. T.I. Kinnunen et al,, "Pregnancy weight gain and breast cancer risk", *BMC Women's Health.* 2004 Oct 21;4(1):7.
30. P. Vaughn, (2002), *Exercise Is Key to Breast Cancer.* Retrieved 20 Feb 2005 from http://www.nih.gov/news/NIH-Record/09_17_2002/story02.htm
31. R.H. Fletcher and K.M. Fairfield, "Vitamins for chronic disease prevention in adults: clinical applications", *JAMA.* 2002 Jun 19;287(23):3127–9
32. T.A. Sellers et al., "Dietary folate intake, alcohol, and risk of breast cancer in a prospective study of postmenopausal women", *Epidemiology.* 2001 Jul;12(4):420–8.
33. M.J. Hill, "Nutrition and human cancer", *Ann N Y Acad Sci.* 1997 Dec 29;833:68–78.
34. ibid.
35. "High levels of animal fat in diet might increase breast cancer risk" (Sep 2003). Retrieved from http://www.breastcancer.org/research_diet_071603.html
36. E. Cho et al., "Premenopausal Fat Intake and Risk of Breast Cancer", *J Natl Cancer Inst.* 2003 Jul 16;95(14):1079–85.
37. I.T.Gram et al., "Breast cancer risk among women who start smoking as teenagers", *Cancer Epidemiol Biomarkers Prev.* 2005 Jan;14(1):61–6.
38. T. Hanaoka et al., "Active and passive smoking and breast cancer risk in middle-aged Japanese women. Int J Cancer. 2005 Mar 20;114(2):317–22.
39. H. Chang et al., "Timing of Breast Surgery, Menstrual Cycle and Prognosis, University of California, San Diego". Retrieved 30 Oct 2004 from http://www.cbcrp.org/research/PageGrantPrintPage.asp?grant_id=241
40. S. Mills and K. Bone, *Principles and practice of phytotherapy*, (London, England: Churchill Livingstone, 2000) pp 354–362.
41. ibid.
42. J.T Pinto and R.S. Rivlin, "Antiproliferative effects of allium derivatives from garlic", *J Nutr.* 2001 Mar;131(3s):1058S–60S.
43. P.J. Hodges and P.C. Kam, "The peri-operative implications of herbal medicines", *Anaesthesia.* 2002 Sep;57(9):889–99.
44. A.T. Borchers et al., "Mushrooms, tumours and immunity", *Proc Soc Exp Biol Med.* 1999;221:281–293
45. M.M. Berger, "Role of trace elements and vitamins in peri-operative nutrition", *Ann Fr Anesth Reanim.* 1995;14 Suppl 2:82–94. French.

46. Food and Nutrition Board, Institute of Medicine, *Vitamin E. Dietary reference intakes for vitamin C, vitamin E, selenium, and carotenoids*, (Washington D.C.: National Academy Press; 2000) pp186–283.
47. ibid.
48. "Carcinogenesis", Metagenics seminar series, New Zealand, Jul/Aug 2001.
49. H. Osieki, *Cancer, a nutritional biochemical approach*, (Queensland, Australia; Bioconcepts, 2002).
50. E. L. Jacobson, "Niacin deficiency and cancer in women", *J Fam Prac*. 2001 50.
51. J. Anastassopoulou and T. Theophanides, "Magnesium-DNA interactions and the possible relation of magnesium to carcinogenesis. Irradiation and free radicals", *Crit Rev Oncol Hematol*. 2002 Apr;42(1):79–91.
52. S. Johnson, "The multifaceted and widespread pathology of magnesium deficiency", *Med Hypotheses*. 2001 Feb;56(2):163–70.
53. Anastassopoulou and Theophanides, loc.sit.
54. T. Hehr et al., "Role of sodium selenite as an adjuvant in radiotherapy of rectal carcinoma" *Med Klin*. 1997 Sep 15;92 Suppl 3:48–9. German.
55. "Carcinogenesis", Metagenics seminar series, New Zealand, Jul/Aug 2001.
56. C. Van Patten, "Coping with taste", *Abreast in the West*. Summer 2002;3:3.
57. Osieki, loc. sit.
58. S. Dreizen et al., "Nutritional deficiencies in patients receiving cancer chemotherapy", *Postgraduate Medicine*. 1990; 87:163–7, 170.
59. J.B. Kirkland, "Niacin and carcinogenesis", *Nutrition and Cancer*. 2003, 46:110.
60. ibid.
61. B.N. Ames, "DNA damage from micronutrient deficiencies is likely to be a major cause of cancer", *Mutat Res*. 2001; 475:7–20.
62. J.C. Spronck, et al., "Chronic DNA damage and niacin deficiency enhance cell injury and cause unusual interactions in NAD and poly (ADP-ribose) metabolism in rat bone marrow", *Nutrition and Cancer*. 2003; 45:124-131.
63. Osieki, loc. sit.
64. Ames, loc. sit.
65. D.D. Kennedy et al., "Low antioxidant vitamin intakes are associated with increases in adverse effects of chemotherapy in children with acute lymphoblastic leukemia", *Am J Clin Nutr*. 2004; 79:1029–36.
66. ibid.
67. B. Nagy, et al., "Chemosensitizing effect of vitamin C in combination with 5-flurouracil in vitro", *In Vivo*. 2003; 17:289–92.
68. J. Drisko, et al., "The use of antioxidants with first line chemotherapy in two cases of ovarian cancer", *J Am Coll Nutr*. 2003; 22:118-23.
69. Ames, loc. sit.
70. A. Pace et al., "Neuroprotective effect of vitamin E supplementation in patients treated with cisplantin chemotherapy", *J Clin Oncol*. 2003; 21: 927-31.
71. H. Lajer and G. Daugaard, "Cisplantin and hypomagnesium", *Cancer Treatment Reviews*. 1999; 25:47–58.
72. C.Y. Guo et al., "Hypomagnesemia associated with chemotherapy in patients treated for acute lymphoblastic leukemia: possible mechanisms", *Oncol Rep*. 2004 Jan;11(1):185–9.

73. Johnson, loc. sit.
74. Anastassopoulou and Theophanides, loc. sit.
75. S. Suresh, "Large-dose intravenous methotrexate-induced cutaneous toxicity: can oral magnesium oxide reduce pain?", *Anesth Analg*. 2003 May;96(5):1413–4.
76. M. Martin et al., "Intravenous and oral magnesium supplementations in the prophylaxis of cisplatin-induced hypomagnesemia. Results of a controlled trial", *Am J Clin Oncol*. 1992 Aug;15(4):348–51.
77. K. El-Bayoumy and R. Sinha, "Mechanisms of mammary cancer chemoprevention by organoselenium compounds", *Mutat Res*. 2004 Jul 13;551(1–2):181–97. Review.
78. R. Sinha and K. El-Bayoumy, "Apoptosis is a critical cellular event in cancer chemoprevention and chemotherapy by selenium compounds", *Curr Cancer Drug Targets*. 2004 Feb;4(1):13–28. Review.
79. S.M. Lippman, "Designing the Selenium and Vitamin E Cancer Prevention Trial (SELECT)" *J Natl Cancer Inst*. 2005 Jan 19;97(2):94–102.
80. A. Federico et al., "Effects of selenium and zinc supplementation on nutritional status in patients with cancer of digestive tract", *Eur J Clin Nutr*. 2001 Apr;55(4):293–7.
81. Y. Beguin et al., "Serum zinc and copper as prognostic factors in acute nonlymphocytic leukemia", *Haematol Blood Transfus*. 1987;30:380–4.
82. O. Falameeva et al., "Macrophage stimulator beta-1-3)-D-carboxymethylglucan improves efficiency of chemotherapy of Lewis lung carcinoma", *Bulletin of Experimental Biology and Medicine*. 2001 Aug;132(8):787–90.
83. G. Kogan et al., "Increased effeciancy of Lewis lung carcinoma chemotherapy with a macrophage stimulator – yeast carboxymethylglucan", *International Pharmacology*. 2002;2:775–81.
84. "Carcinogenesis", Metagenics seminar series, New Zealand, Jul/Aug 2001.
85. "HRT: What are women (and their doctors) to Do?", *The Lancet*. 2004;364(9451):5000
86. M.E. Bracke et al., "Influence of tangeretin on tamoxifen's therapeutic benefit in mammary cancer", *J Natl Cancer Inst* 1999;91:354–9.
87. F.S. Kenny et al., "Gamma linolenic acid with tamoxifen as primary therapy in breast cancer", *Int J Cancer* 2000;85:643–8.
88. N. Guthrie et al., "Inhibition of proliferation of oestrogen receptor-negative MDA-MB-435 and -positive MCF-7 human breast cancer cells by palm oil tocotrienols and tamoxifen, alone and in combination", *J Nutr* 1997;127:544S–8S.
89. K. Lockwood, et al., "Apparent partial remission of breast cancer in 'high risk' patients supplemented with nutritional antioxidants, essential fatty acids and coenzyme Q10", *Mol Aspects Med*. 1994;15 Suppl:s231–40.
90. K. Folkers, "Relevance of the biosynthesis of CoQ10 and four bases of DNA as a rationale for the molecular causes of cancer and a therapy", *Biochem Biophys Res Commun*. 1996;224:358–61.
91. Lockwood, loc. sit.
92. K. Lockwood et al., "Progress on therapy of breast cancer with vitamin Q10 and the regression of metastases", *Biochem Biophys Res Commun*. 1995 Jul 6;212(1):172–7

93. D. Spiegel, *Living Beyond Limits*, (New York: Ballantine Books, 1993).
94. M. Watson et al., "Influence of psychological response on survival in breast cancer: a population-based cohort study", *Lancet*. 1999, Oct 16;354;9187.
95. Cancer Society of New Zealand, *Living With Cancer – What Do I Tell The Children?* (Wellington: 2001).
96. National Health & Medical Research Council, *Psychosocial Clinical Practice Guidelines*, (Canberra: 1999) p.38.
97. G. E. Westberg, *Good Grief: A Constructive Approach to the Problem of Loss*, (Augsburg Fortress Publishers, 1979).
98. J. Link, *Take Charge of Your Breast Cancer*, (New York: Owl Books, 2002) (13):32
99. P.E. Hansen et al., "Personality Traits, Health Behavior, and Risk for Cancer: A Prospective Study of a Swedish Twin Cohort", *Cancer*: January 24, 2005.
100. Link, op. sit. p 147.
101. J.R. Harris et al., *Diseases of the Breast*, 3rd Edn, (Lippincott Williams & Wilkins, 2004) p 1457.
102. K. Lillberg et al., "Stressful life events and risk of breast cancer in 10,808 women: a cohort study", *Am J Epidemiol* 2003 Mar 1;157(5):415–23
103. New Zealand Cancer Society of New Zealand, *Sexuality and Cancer*, (Wellington: 2003) p 22.
104. C. H. van Gils et al., "Consumption of Vegetables and Fruits and Risk of Breast Cancer", *J Am Med Assoc*. Jan 12, 2005; 293:183–193.
105. S.A. Smith-Warner et al., "Intake of fruits and vegetables and risk of breast cancer: a pooled analysis of cohort studies", *JAMA*. 2001 Feb 14;285(6):769–76.
106. E. Riboli and T. Norat, "Epidemiologic evidence of the protective effect of fruit and vegetables on cancer risk", *Am J Clin Nutr*. 2003 Sep;78(3 Suppl):559S–569S.
107. A.S. Malin et al., "Intake of fruits, vegetables and selected micronutrients in relation to the risk of breast cancer", *Int J Cancer*. 2003 Jun 20;105(3):413–8.
108. L. Kenton, *The Powerhouse Diet*, (London: Random House, 2004).
109. K. Mokbel, "Risk-reducing strategies for breast cancer – a review of recent literature", *Int J Fertil Womens Med*. 2003 Nov–Dec;48(6):274–7.
110. U. Erasmus, *Fats that heal, fats that kill*, 2nd Edn. (Canada: Alive Books, 1996) p 273.
111. ibid.
112. M.S. Brignall, "Prevention and treatment of cancer with indole-3-carbinol", *Altern Med Rev*. 2001 Dec;6(6):580–9. Review.
113. K. Dedyna, "Iodine: Bosom Buddy", *Victoria Times Colonist*, Sept 9, 1997:D1
114. J. Mann and E. Aitken, "The re-emergence of iodine deficiency in New Zealand?", *J NZ Med Assoc*. 14 March 2003;116(1170).
115. ibid.
116. J.R. Weiss et al., "Epidemiology of male breast cancer", *Cancer Epidemiol Biomarkers Prev*. 2005 Jan;14(1):20–6.
117. O. Warburg, "On the origin of cancer cells", *Science*. 1956 Feb;123:309–14.
118. T. Volk et al., "pH in human tumor xenografts: effect of intravenous administration of glucose", *Br J Cancer*. 1993 Sep;68(3):492–500.

119. M. Digirolamo, *Diet and cancer: markers, prevention and treatment*, (New York: Plenum Press, 1994) p 203.
120. D.B. Leeper et al., "Effect of i.v. glucose versus combined i.v. plus oral glucose on human tumor extracellular pH for potential sensitization to thermoradiotherapy", *Int J Hyperthermia*. 1998 May–Jun;143:257–69.
121. L.S. Augustin et al., "Dietary glycaemic index and glycaemic load, and breast cancer risk: a case-control study", *Ann Oncol*. 2001;12(11):1533–1538.
122. C.R. Jonas et al., "Dietary glycaemic index, glycaemic load, and risk of incident breast cancer in postmenopausal women", *Cancer Epidemiol Biomarkers Prev*. 2003;12(6):573–577.
123. D.S. Michaud et al., "Dietary sugar, glycaemic load, and pancreatic cancer risk in a prospective study", *J Natl Cancer Inst*. 2002;94(17):1293–1300.
124. L.S. Augustin et al., "Dietary glycaemic index, glycaemic load and ovarian cancer risk: a case-control study in Italy", *Ann Oncol*. 2003;14(1):78–84.
125. L.S. Augustin et al., "Glycaemic index and glycaemic load in endometrial cancer", *Int J Cancer*. 2003;105(3):404–407.
126. S. Franceschi et al., "Dietary glycaemic load and colorectal cancer risk", *Ann Oncol*. 2001;12(2):173–178.
127. J. Ratcliff, *Low carb made easy*, (Victoria, Australia: Hinkler Books, 2002).
128. D.T. Sava and G. Duwe, "Oestrogenic and antiproliferative properties of genistein and other flavonoids in human breast cancer cells in vitro", *Nutrition and Cancer*. 1997;27:31–40.
129. K. Jaga and H. Duvvi, "Risk reduction for DDT toxicity and carcinogenesis through dietary modification", *J Reprod Soc Health* 2001;121 (2):107–113.
130. S. Barnes, "Phyto-oestrogens and breast cancer", *Phyto-oestrogens, Bailliere's Clinical Endocrinology and Metabolism*, ed. H. Adlercreutz (Bailliere Tindal, 1998) pp 605–624.
131. Sava and Duwe, loc.sit.
132. C.Y. Hsieh, et al, "Oestrogenic effects on genistein on the growth of oestrogen receptor-positive human breast cancer (MCF-7) cells in vitro an in vivo", *Cancer Research*. 1998; 58:3833–3838.
133. Breast Cancer Fund and Breast Cancer Action, "State of the evidence. What is the connection between the environment and breast cancer", 3rd Edn, ed N. Evans. (San Francisco, USA, 2004) pp 28–29.
134. ibid.
135. J. Dorn, "Lifetime Physical Activity and Breast Cancer Risk in Pre- and Postmenopausal Women", *Medicine & Science in Sports & Exercise*. 2003, Feb; 35(2).
136. Nkondjock and Ghadirian, loc. sit.
137. *Breast Cancer Facts* (1 Oct 2003). Retrieved 16 Feb 2005 from "The New Zealand Breast Cancer Foundation" http://www.nzbcf.org.nz/news/display.asp?itemId=190
138. J.R. Weiss et al., "Epidemiology of male breast cancer", *Cancer Epidemiol Biomarkers Prev*. 2005 Jan;14(1):20–6.
139. ibid.
140. J. Blue et al., "Overview of breast cancer prevention – a search for the causes of breast cancer", *NZ GP Mag*. 1998 Oct;32–35.

141. ibid.
142. ibid.
143. ibid.
144. "Laboratory assessments. Women's hormonal health assessment". Retrieved on 6 Mar 2005 from "Great Smokies Diagnostic Lab" http://www.gsdl.com/home/assessments/womenshealth/
145. C.O. Simonton et al., *Getting Well Again: The Bestselling Classic About the Simontons' Revolutionary Lifesaving Self-Awareness Techniques,* (New York: Bantam Books, Reissue edition, 1992).
146. C.O. Simonton, *The Healing Journey,* (Authors Choice Press, 2002).
147. Link, op. cit., pp 127–129.
148. *Patch Adams*, the film, Universal Studios, 1998
149. L. S. Berk et al,. Loma Linda, *The Scientist: The News Journal for the Life Scientist,* October 2, 2000
150. S. Gawain, *Creative Visualisation,* (New World Books, 1978).
151. ibid. Part 2:(41):81.
152. ibid. Part 1:(1):27.
153. M. Hernandez-Reif et al., "Breast cancer patients have improved mmune and neuroendocrine functions following massage therapy", *J Psychosom Res.* 2004 Jul;57(1):45–52.
154. C. B. Pert, *Molecules of Emotion,* (Simon & Schuster, 1997).
155. *China Reflexology Symposium Report,* China Reflexology Association, 1996.
156. Retrieved 24 Mar 2005 from http://www.wisechoices.com
157. H. Murad with D. Partie Lange, *Wrinkle-Free Forever, The 5-Minute, 5-Week Dermatologist's Program,* (New York: St Martin's Griffin Press, 2003).
158. Retrieved on 19 Nov 2004 from http://www.breastcancer.org

Bibliography

Berger, K. and Bostwick, J. *A Woman's Decision: breast care, treatment and reconstruction.* St Louis: Quality Medical Publishing, Inc., 1999.

Ellis, K. *Shattering the cancer myth.* Victoria: Hinkler Books, 2003.

Gawain, S. *Creative Visualisation.* California: New World Library, 1995.

Kenton, L. *The Power House Diet.* UK: Random House, 2004.

Link, J. et al. *The Breast Cancer Survival Manual: A Step-By-Step Guide for the Woman With Newly Diagnosed Breast Cancer.* 3rd Rev Edn. New York: Owl Books, 2003.

Lopez, L. *Natural Health: an A to Z Guide.* Auckland: David Bateman Ltd, 2004.

Love, S. and Lindsey, K. *Dr Susan Love's Breast Book.* 3rd Edn. Cambridge, MA: Perseus Publishing, 2000.

Malloy, A. *Get A Life – simple strategies for work/life balance.* Auckland: Random House, 2004.

Mills, S. and Bone, K. *Principles and practice of phytotherapy.* London: Churchill Livingstone, 2000.

Pizzorno, J. and Murray, M. *Textbook of natural medicine.* 2nd Edn. Edinburgh: Churchill Livingstone, 2000.

Radd, S. and Setchell, K. *Eat to live.* Auckland: Hodder Moa Beckett, 2000.

Ratcliff, J. *Low carb made easy.* Victoria: Hinkler books, 2002.

Stoppard, M. *Woman's Body – A Manual for Life.* London: Dorling Kindersley, 1999.

Index

5HTP 63

acidophilus 47, 72, 73
acupressure 109
acupuncture 109
affirmations 109, 110, 111
age 31, 33
alcohol 29, 34, 86
aloe vera 50; juice 47, 49, 50, 55
Anastrozole (Arimidex) 56; side effects 57
animal fat 34, 85
antioxidants 89, 96, 99
anxiety medication 24
areola 17
aromatherapy 108, 109
atypical hyperplasia (AH) 33
Auckland Cancer Society 60
axilla 69
axillary lymph nodes 18

B complex multi 64
B vitamins 99
Bach™ Flower 64, 66
balance 114
beans 97
Beta 1.3 Glucan 54, 55
bifidus 72, 73
bilateral mastectomy 40
biopsy 23, 24
birth control pills 30, 32
black cohosh 74
borage oils 57
bovine cartilage 43
brachytherapy 48
breast cancer 25, 26; *in situ* 26
breast conservation surgery 40
breast forms 124
breast lumps 20, 33
breast self-examination 19
breast tumours 25
breasts 17, 18

calcium 64
Californian poppy 64
calorie restriction 90
CAM 38, 39, 42
Cancer Society 28
carotenoids 83, 90
cereals 97

cervical lymph nodes 18
chemo brain 53
chemotherapy 48, 50–53
child bearing 32
children 61, 62
citrus bioflavonoids 57
cleavers 70
cloves 43
coenzyme Q10 58, 94, 96
complex carbohydrates 63
connective tissue hyperplasia 20
contraceptive hormones 32
core biopsy 24; stereotactic 24
counselling 60
creative visualisation 109, 110
cysteine 90
cysts 20, 21

dairy 97
deodorant 49
depression 62, 63, 64
diet 29, 81, 96
dietary fibre 83
digestive enzymes 55
diindolylmethane (DIM) 72, 87, 96
dithiolthiones 83
dong quai 74
ductal carcinoma *in situ* (DCIS) 26, 33
ductal system 18

echinacea 44
endogenous oestrogen 30
endorphins 107
Epsom salts 71
essential fatty acids (EFA) 85
evening primrose oil 43, 57, 85
exercise 29, 34, 46, 47, 70, 79, 97, 98, 127
exicisional surgical biopsy 24
exogenous oestrogen 30

family history 31
fatigue 64, 65
fats 85
fertility 67
feverfew 43
fibre 84; supplements 47
fibroadenomas 20
fine aspiration 24
fish oil 43, 96
flavonoid 90

flax seed 87; oil 86, 96
folic acid 83, 99
fruit 82, 83, 97

garlic 43, 44
gender 31
genetic predisposition 31
genetics 29
ginger 43
ginkgo 43
ginseng 43, 44, 64
glucose 91
glucosinolates 83
glutamine 55
glutathione 55
glycaemic index (GI) 91
goitrogenic effect 93
goldenseal 43
grapefruit juice 43
green tea 102
grief 65
guilt 66

hair 116
herbal detoxes 96
herbal extracts 70
herbs 43
Herceptin 56
Hodgkin's disease 32
homeopathic liquid arnica 46
hormonal treatments 56
hormone fluctuations 20
hormone replacement therapy (HRT) 30, 32, 103, 104
hormone sensitive cancers 56
HRT see hormone replacement therapy

immune multi 44, 46
indentation 26
indole-3-carbinol 83, 87, 102
infertility 51
inflammation 21
inflammatory breast cancer 26
infraclavicular lymph nodes 18
intraoperative radiotherapy 48
invasive (infiltrating) ductal carcinoma *in situ* (IDC) 26
invasive (infiltrating) lobular carcinoma *in situ* (ILC) 26
iodine 89
ionising radiation 99
iron 64

143

isoflavones 72, 73, 102

kelp 96
kudzu 73

lactation 18
laughter 106
legumes 97, 102
lignans 88, 102
liquorice 43
lobular carcinoma *in situ* (LCIS) 26, 33
lobules 18
Look Good Feel Better 115, 117, 120
lump 26
lumpectomy 40
lumpiness 20
lymph 68
lymph node 18, 25, 68, 69
lymphatic massage 70
lymphatic system 68
lymphocytes 25
lymphoedema 68, 69

magnesium 49, 50, 54, 55, 64
Magnetic Resonance Imaging 23
makeup 120
mammary glands 18
mammogram 21
mammosite 48
manganese 90
massage 111
mastalgia (breast pain) 20
mastectomy 40
meditation 111, 112
medullary carcinoma 26
menopausal symptoms 73, 74
menopause 32, 71
menstruation 20, 29, 32
metastatic disease 27
methionine 90
milk production 18
minerals 45, 96; formula 96; supplements 94
Montgomery glands 17
motherwort 74
MRI see Magnetic Resonance Imaging
mucinous carcinoma 26
multi vitamins 45, 94, 96
mushroom extracts 44

Nat Mur (sodium chloride) 70
Nat Sulph (sodium sulphate) 70
naturopath 38
nipple discharge 20, 21
nipples 17
nutrition 34
nuts 96, 102

obesity 33, 90, 127
oestradiol 71
oestrogen 29, 30, 71, 72, 73, 84, 87, 102, 127
Oestrogen Metabolism Assessment 73, 93, 103
oils 96
omega 3 49, 63, 85, 86, 102
omega 6 85, 86
oral contraceptives 30, 103
ovarian cancer 53

Paget's disease of the nipple 27
passionflower 64
Phyllodes tumour 27
phyto-oestrogens 72, 73, 84, 88, 102
plant oestrogens see phyto-oestrogens
prebiotic formulas 55
pregnancies 29
pregnancy-related breast cancer 68
prosthesis 124
protein 63, 97; powders 55
Psychoneuro-immunology 105

race 31
radiation 29, 99, 100; burns 50; therapy 47
radiotherapy 47, 48, 49
radium nosode 49
raw food 82, 83
recommended daily intake (RDI) 94, 95, 96
reconstruction 41, 42
red clover 43, 44, 73
reflexology 112, 113
reiki 113
relationships 77
Rescue Remedy 45, 46, 66
risk factors 30, 35
rosemary 72, 88

sage 74
saturated fat 85
scarring 47
screening methods 22
sea salt 71
seaweed 88, 102
seeds 96, 102
selenium 49, 50, 54, 55, 90, 99
self heal 70
sentinel node biopsy 40
serotonin 63
sex 78
shark cartilage 43
side effects 52
skin 117
sleep 114
smoking 34, 98, 99, 127
soy 73, 92, 93, 97
soy foods 72, 73
spirulina 47, 65
St John's wort 43, 64
stress 75
sugar 91
sulforaphane 83, 87, 102
supplements 39, 43, 44, 50, 57, 72, 94, 96
support 39
supraclavicular lymph nodes 18
surgery 28, 40, 42, 43
sweet clover 70

Tamoxifen 56; side effects 57
the pill 103
thermography 23
tissue cell salts 64, 70
tocotrienols 58
tubular carincoma 26

ultrasound 22
UV radiation 100

vaginal dryness 78, 79
valerian 43
vegetables 82, 83, 87, 97
vitamin B3 (niacin) 49, 50, 53, 55
vitamin C 53, 55, 83, 90, 99
vitamin E 43, 45, 46, 53, 55, 83
vitamins 96

weight gain 52, 75
wild yam 73
wire localisation biopsy 24

xeno-oestrogens 30
x-rays 99

yoga 113, 114

zinc 54, 55, 90